Cut Out The Bullshit

There's Always Another Way

Shim Ravalia

ii

Cut Out The Bullshit

© 2024 **Shim Ravalia**

ISBN: 9781738434800 Paperback

Published by: Inspired By Publishing

Cover Designed By: Tanya Grant, The TNG Designs Group Limited

The strategies in this book are presented primarily for enjoyment and educational purposes. Every effort has been made to trace copyright holders and obtain their permission for the use of copyright material.

The information and resources provided in this book are based upon the authors' personal experiences. Any outcome, income statements or other results, are based on the authors' experiences and there is no guarantee that your experience will be the same. There is an inherent risk in any business enterprise or activity and there is no guarantee that you will have similar results as the author as a result of reading this book.

The author reserves the right to make changes and assumes no responsibility or liability whatsoever on behalf of any purchaser or reader of these materials.

Acknowledgements

Firstly, I want to thank my great friend, my mentor and my business partner Chloë Bisson. Without her love and support and how much she inspired me with her first book as well as the little nudge in the ribs, I would never have had the inspiration to put this book together and get the message out there.

Secondly, a massive thank you to all my beautiful clients who have continued to inspire me, teach me and for their trust, love and support in helping me put this book together.

And lastly, to my brilliant gut health team past and present who have been just amazing throughout the whole process and I am so grateful to work with them in getting this book the attention it deserves, helping people get to optimal health and pushing The Gut Intuition to new heights.

I am truly grateful forever.

Foreword

Shim Ravalia is a beacon of wisdom and empowerment. Her no-nonsense book "Cut Out The Bullshit" is a beacon of truth, so prepare to embark on a transformative journey towards optimal health and well-being.

Shim and I actually met when the world paused and became chaotic. We connected through a group of other like-minded women in business and we talked and talked for ages about health and the conversations happened at the right time as I was reevaluating my own health.

This isn't just another health book; it's a life-changing compass that guides you through the maze of nutrition, decoding the enigmatic microbiome and unlocking the keys to vitality. Shim Ravalia's words are truly engaging; each chapter is a treasure trove of actionable insights.

Shim doesn't hold back; she lays it all bare with honesty and heartwarming candour. Her wisdom isn't just theoretical; it's born from real-life experiences, the lives she's touched and the tears she's shared.

In a world obsessed with upgrading gadgets, isn't it time we upgraded ourselves? "Cut Out The Bullshit" is your ticket to a new mindset that recognises the profound connection between what you consume and your overall wellness.

Prepare to be captivated by the fascinating realm of gut health. Shim Ravalia invites you on a self-discovery expedition within your body's inner ecosystem. This book isn't just informative; it's your guiding compass towards a healthier you. As Shim wisely puts it, "You are not what you eat... You are what you absorb, digest, and excrete."

I'm thrilled to introduce you to this indispensable resource. Get ready to transform your life, unlock your true potential, and embrace the vibrant, healthier you that's been waiting to emerge. Because it's time to take control of your health, one bite at a time. Happy reading!

Sharon Roberts
Entertainment and Business Consultant

Dedication

I want to dedicate this book to Mum and Dad. To Mum, the "Iron Lady" of our family, who showed me to never give up no matter what, keep moving forward and keep my head up high. To Dad for being the true hero of our family. For teaching me so much about life, health and connection. You are no longer here today however, you are always forever in my heart.

Table of Contents

Introduction: It's Not Sexy 1

Chapter 1: Just Like That 7

Chapter 2: Doing Everything & Achieving Nothing...15

Chapter 3: World War 3..29

Chapter 4: The Gut..35

Chapter 5: Gut Health And Stress 47

Chapter 6: Gut Health And Sugar 51

Chapter 7: Gut Health And Sleep....................................61

Chapter 8: Gut Health And Hydration...........................73

Chapter 9: Gut Health And Movement 81

Chapter 10: Gut Health And Your Environment.........87

Chapter 11: What Is Your Body Really Telling You?.101

Chapter 12: Why Does Disconnect Happen?..............107

Chapter 13: The Link Between Depression And Gut
Health 113

Chapter 14: Work Life Balance Is BS!...........................119

Chapter 15: Not One But Two...127

Conclusion: Is The Clock Ticking?.............................. 137

About the Author 139

References and Resources 141

Introduction

It's Not Sexy

Creating changes in your life, career, business, health is often not sexy work at all most of the time. Change is hard because you have to deal with your ego freaking out, triggers that pop up left, right and center and you are constantly absorbing all sorts of information thrown at you in your environment every day. You want to feel safe and comfortable therefore any sort of change becomes quite frankly, uncomfortable as fuck.

What's not really taught in the mainstream health space much is that it's actually a really positive sign that you are uncomfortable when it comes to change because you are simply asked to upgrade your way of thinking and how you are treating your body because you are capable of potentially so much more. Too often I see, hear and feel coaches, mentors, gurus, experts, specialists, doctors, consultants, the influencers on Instagram, that lunatic who's taken the 3 day life coaching, nutrition course online posting their certificate telling the world that they are now an 'expert' and that they can help you and fix all your problems that work on your mindset and all will be well, take this supplement and it will fix your problems, get this injection and it won't come back.

This is one of the dangers of today…

So, my work and purpose as a gut stress expert isn't sexy work. I do not have people come and work with me because they fancied exploring looking at their own shit. Far from it. These are the individuals who have tried everything and have gotten nowhere, still in pain, sick and tired of feeling sick and tired, not heard, feel like they are disappearing and have worries through the roof. Don't just take my word for it, you'll be reading about real life case studies of individuals who decided that enough was enough and have come out of the other side of it. I've shared exactly how I helped them and why and I hope it helps you in some way to look at things differently too.

You've got to accept that in order for you to have a different outcome with your health, a different outcome with your business with your finances, a different outcome with your career etc, you've got to reboot and upgrade your systems. Too many people try to operate like Windows 11 while their mindset, attitude, and systems are operating on Windows 5. I've used Windows as an example here because I'm not an Apple fan! Haha!

You will notice that this book is packed with lots of tips that have been backed by Science and from my own experience on how to really cut out the bullshit and start to improve your health literally from today. I want you to use this book as a starting point in rebooting and upgrading your system of thinking, your attitude and your approach towards your own health. Whether you believe it or not, you have a purpose here and without health on your side, it's going to be a long and messy road. The fact that you've picked this book up to read tells me that there is a level of readiness, albeit a subtle one, that you are somewhat curious and ready to hear more of what I've got to say and you do take responsibility for yourself and your own actions.

Well, you are in the right place!

I also want to say clearly that where you are today with your health and life is not entirely your fault either. You've been fed a lot of crap along the way, you've been shamed and judged in society without even realising it and been gaslighted by some doctors and specialists. You've been very hard on yourself to strive more without anyone ever telling you anything differently or just supporting you. So therefore, I want this book to be your support, your go-to guide for taking back control of your own health that has been evidently snatched away from you before your very own eyes by these so-called experts I mentioned earlier. In this book, I have shared real life examples of some incredible human beings who were once not in a great place but took the journey to heal themselves inside and out and I've shared exactly how they did it. Please do not attempt to try anything shared in some of these case studies by yourself before actually speaking to a professional expert. Why? Because everything I share with you in this book has been personalised to that individual.

My intention with this book is to give you a simple structure to follow that works for you and for you only. This is the magic that makes it work! Change is the only thing that is constant in your life so you can't avoid it but you can certainly learn and grow from it. My favourite part of this journey of change? To have fun and play with it because there is a higher chance of those changes sticking around for a lot longer.

These are my core values with life, health and business:

Change
Learn & Grow
Play

And if these core values resonate with you in this book then I give you full permission to grab them with both hands and explore it for yourself.

Disclaimer: I'm not here to reinvent the wheel and claim to be a doctor and tell you I can cure all diseases. I am all about meeting you where you are at and where you want to be and closing that gap with tools and resources that work for you and for you only so that you are no longer guessing, assuming, wondering and trying to figure it all out by yourself. You are not meant to hence why The Gut Intuition exists and why I created this book in the first place. Prevention is better than cure.

I've got your back...

So, are you ready?

Chapter 1

Just Like That

It was Tuesday 12th June 2018 and I arrived at the A & E as quickly as I could. It was around 11pm in the night and I walked through the automatic doors and that typical hospital smell instantly hit me alongside busy doctors and nurses working hard to care for patients in need.

I could hear all the machines beeps and sounds going off as well as the walls of the A & E covered with charts and information against the plain white walls. The floors almost had this sheen look on them as I looked down walking along this long corridor to find my mum and dad.

You see an hour before, my dad got really sick and had vomited quietly. My mum didn't hear a thing until she went to check up on him and to her horror, he didn't look well and was struggling to breathe as he was almost choking on his own vomit. I quickly called the ambulance and they could hear him on the phone struggling to breathe and within a few minutes were at our door ready to take him into A & E.

I entered this room where I saw my dad lying down helplessly and desperately trying to breathe but his eyes were closed the whole time. His breathing sounded like something was really stuck inside his body and sounded rough and edgy. He had all sorts of stickers stuck on his chest to keep an eye on him. I remember saying his name and I could see he wanted to open his eyes but he just couldn't anymore. My intuition was telling me that he was shutting down, yet I remained hopeful for the sake of my mum and the fact that I didn't even want to admit or even imagine that I could be losing my dad. For me, it was the case of getting Dad well again, the Doctors will give their medications and we can all go home together again. Mum was at this point frantically pacing up and down the room feeling worried, nervous and just not sure what's really going on.

A young female doctor came into the room and said hello to me and my mum. She seemed fairly polite and just doing her job as a doctor would do. I remember her face being quite expressionless and just neutral, checking the monitors, the chart board and my dad's breathing.

I remember standing there with my arms crossed looking up at the ceiling and waiting for the Doctor to come over and just explain what's going on and then we can all make a plan of action and go home.

I'll never forget what happened next and the exact words this doctor had said to me.

"So, your Dad doesn't have long left. It might be a good idea for you to start calling close family members to say their goodbye".

It didn't quite register for me. I repeated back to the doctor what I thought she just told me because I felt I may have heard it wrong. It was right and he didn't have long left.

The doctor left the room and a tsunami of emotions just took over me. I burst into tears and felt so out of control and hopeless to watch him breathe his final breath and I was standing there and not able to help him in any way. I felt my mum's hand on the right side of my shoulder and I turned around and by the look on my face and the tears of sadness rolling down my cheeks, she knew what was happening yet she needed me to explain what the doctor had said.

As the minutes went by one by one and the hours started to creep on, more and more close family members came as quickly as they could to be with my dad in his final hours of being on earth. He was still holding on, trying to take a deep breath in and out with his eyes firmly closed. I do believe he was still able to feel everyone's presence there and just didn't want to leave just yet.

It was now Wednesday 13th June 2018 and it was around 6.30am in the morning. My mum had forgotten a few things at home that she needed for my dad so she had me and my sister go home to quickly grab the things and come back asap. I was around 2 minutes away from my house and I received a phone call from my brother asking us to come back as Dad was slowly leaving now. His breathing had slowed down and was quite shallow and he was slowly losing the fight to stay alive now. His body was just shutting down.

I quickly turned my car around and drove to the hospital with my sister as quickly as I could. I remember it being a really sunny day without a cloud in sight and the streets just being really quiet at that time of the morning. Yet the journey back to the hospital was an interesting one. With the streets being quiet and hardly any pedestrians around, I hit every red traffic light going there. I was getting more and more frustrated because all I wanted to do was to just say my final goodbyes to my dad and everything seemed to be stopping or delaying me from doing so as it certainly felt like it at the time. I even had a passenger cross the road out of nowhere on a green traffic light which delayed things even more.

I got to the hospital and I was too late. He had left already and they had already moved him to another room so that everyone could privately say their goodbyes. I remember walking to the door and entering a room full of tears, crying, pain. It was harrowing.

By this point, I was nervous, I felt pain and numb at the same time and all of a sudden saying goodbye became one of the hardest things to do at that moment. There he was lying down, all covered up with blankets no longer struggling fighting to stay alive. He looked at peace and I leaned down slowly and gave him a kiss on his right cheek and said goodbye. He was still warm at this point. I took a deep breath and took a step back to let others say their goodbyes too.

Coming back home that morning felt really surreal. I walked through the front door and the home felt empty with people in it. I walked into the living room where Dad used to sleep because he lost the use of his legs so it was a lot easier for him to just stay downstairs. I glanced over to his bed where the covers still had creases in them from when he last slept on it. His bottle of water was still on the table half-drunk with a straw in it and his clothes were by the washing machine. It was a very surreal feeling that less than 24 hours ago, he was alive and now he wasn't and never ever was going to be either. It was a difficult thought to come to terms with and accept that day and a hard one to process because everything happened so quickly and dramatically changed and shaped my life from there onwards. So much of that day he had passed was a blur for me because it was a shock and quite traumatic to unexpectedly lose my dad just like that. You see, six months before, My Dad's specialist told him that he had half a year to live which was a real shock to the whole family. My parents then decided to get a second opinion and this particular specialist said the opposite, that he still had many years ahead of him still and that he was doing pretty good with a brain tumour. We had two very different opinions and I guess the first one was right. The last thing I remember is being in my parents room hugging my mum on the bed who was crying, completely in shock and distraught of losing her husband of 45 years just like that. I hugged her till she got tired of crying and fell asleep.

Here's what I learnt about grief itself: There isn't this manual telling you how to grieve a loss of someone or something that was close to you and nor should there be. Grief is such a powerful individual journey of lessons and healing if you choose to look at it that way.

I had some really deep thoughts about how I was never going to see my dad again on my birthday every January, a good morning or a good night, to be there on my wedding day if I ever got married or be the grandad to my children if I ever had children, or go on holiday with him and make beautiful memories.

My dad's departure from this world forced me to question my own happiness which was actually a really positive experience despite the grief and the loss I was going through at the time.

What is it that makes me really happy, I mean truly fulfilled?

What do I want to dedicate my time and energy into that's fun, creative and that I look forward to every single time?

How do I want to feel in my own skin everyday?

What is the next business I want to run?

What kind of lifestyle do I want to live unapologetically?

What sort of legacy do I want to leave when I die?

I remember sitting in my living room during this time, quite spaced out and these intuitive questions coming through and really opening myself to be aware of these questions that I believe my higher self at the time was guiding me to lean towards. I didn't have the answers to these questions straight away yet I was aware that they were coming up for me and I needed to take notice and sit with them for a while as after all, I was just aimlessly living day to day without a goal in sight.

Chapter 2

Doing Everything & Achieving Nothing

March 2012 was a super proud moment for me. I couldn't quite believe that I had my own business now and that I was an owner of a company. I loved the thrill of it because it was something brand new, something that I had created on my terms, my rules and my way.

The first three years of my business I simply ran it by myself with no staff. My mindset at the time was just to save as much money as I could so that I could pay myself on time every month. Financial security has always been a big deal for me and still is. I wore all the hats you could have when running a business and looking back at my journey, I sometimes wonder how I really managed everything by myself. I was the marketing manager, the finance manager, looking after the social media channels, looking at budgets, overheads, content calendar, the admin, taking the business to the next level, looking after every single client I had and more coming in. I had multitasking mastered down to an art. I was so good at it. But most of the time, it was exhausting and if I didn't do it, there would have been a backlog of admin to catch up on every day and admin is boring.

I spent a lot of time in my first few years working all the hours to make the business a success; success being money at the time. What was put across to me in the business world in so many different ways was I had to hustle to get to where I needed to get to, I had to work hard and play hard and fake it till you make it which is the worse advice someone gave me once to which I never really took any notice of. Come to think of it, these behaviours did serve me because it pushed me to take more action in my business.

One cold January evening, I sat down alone in my bedroom dreading to just look at my bank account because deep down my intuition was just telling me something was off. Nevertheless, I logged in and realised I had 76 pence left in my account. My heart sank, my mind was racing and my inner critical voice got louder and louder. I worked so hard and I was damn busy with clients but it didn't quite reflect this on what was in my bank account at the time. I honestly felt like a failure. At times, I would cringe at the thought of when someone would ask me how my business was going. I'd always reply back "it's going really well thanks" with a smile on my face knowing full well that wasn't the case many times. I was very good at hiding the pain and internalising my stress. I wouldn't advise this approach at all.

Doing everything and achieving nothing is what was so loud in my head at the time. Of course, when something doesn't work anymore, it's time to look at things differently and do it differently too.

2015 is where I looked at things differently, I got myself a business coach who showed the right systems, teams and processes to have in place to ensure success in your business. At last, business was working well again and honestly I was obsessed with my results and I wanted to achieve more and more and I loved what was coming into my bank account and I loved the team that I was growing as well which meant more holidays, weekends offs and focused work on the business and not in the business all of the time.

As 2017 approached, I naturally started to look at how I helped people a little bit differently. I always wondered why a client who was pain free from seeing me after 3 months would come back again in more pain than before and almost start their treatment plan all over again? I could feel myself navigating more into the depths of human emotions and how they manifest as symptoms in our body and in this book, I will share some resources for you to go and geek out on too.

The more I went down the rabbit hole of the emotion code, the more I was falling in love with it and falling out of love with Sports Therapy. It just wasn't satisfying enough anymore just looking at physical health but not also looking into emotional and mental health too. It felt incomplete to me and I just knew that this was the path I wanted to take to help more people. After all, it's an absolutely fascinating area of the human experience.

January 2018 is where I made a bold move to move away from my Sports Therapy clinic and move more into holistic coaching of some sort; I wasn't sure what, how, where I just knew that is what needed to be done. However, life had other plans for me along the way where not only did my dad pass away that same year but by the end of 2018, my health was in horrendous shape. The burning sensation inside my stomach progressively got worse and worse, I hardly slept and looked dreadful when I looked at myself in the mirror every morning. I put on weight which I held a lot of shame and guilt about since I was in the health and fitness industry showing others how to be fit and healthy. I just wanted to hide away in a hole and not come out. That's how I honestly felt most days. I just wasn't enjoying life and I was deeply unhappy within myself. I reacted to a lot of foods and I love flavourful foods and I felt no joy in cutting things out or eating bland foods because after spice is life and I grew up on spices, and herbs.

The one core decision I needed to make was I had to put my health first. I had put creating another business to the side for now and just focused on getting better because I was going down a slippery slope of ill health if I didn't sort these issues out right now. There is never a good time to start working on your health; you work on your health everyday.

I initially went down the NHS root in 2017 when my stomach issues were getting louder and it did not help me. It was a disappointing experience where the Doctor at the time asked me a few questions whilst writing a prescription of Gaviscon which is medication to treat stomach upset, heartburn and indigestion. Looking back, it was probably IBS at this stage but progressed to something a lot worse later on. From here onwards, I did the best that I could for this issue with the tools and resources I had at the time. However, coming to the end of 2018 and going down the functional medicine route and doing a deeper analysis and testing in stomach issues, it appeared that I had a bacterial infection called Klebsiella Oxytoca for around four years that I didn't even know I had. It left me scratching my head for a while. I mean how could I miss an infection to this scale that was right under my nose?

Well, I didn't know what I didn't know at the time and it was all very new to me and quite exciting too. To get to the bottom of my symptoms and to factor in everything that I was going through with the grief and loss, weight gain, confidence issues to my mindset - THIS WAS A GAME CHANGER!

I was hooked now and I can honestly say that it was my mess with my own health that created my message for you today and this was also the spark that created my second company called The Gut Intuition.

It is because of my own journey that I was able to help individuals like Gita.

Gita got in touch with us in August 2021 because she was really struggling with fatigue, bloating, stomach cramps and gas after eating meals. She was struggling to digest fats, was suffering with headaches and had poor sleep as she was waking up in the middle of the night and had sugar cravings. Due to the nature of her business, she was quite stressed and was overthinking a lot about work related projects etc at night so she couldn't really switch off most of the time, even at the weekends. Gita was a business owner (still is) and she was working long hours with little to no support at that time. She was working on the weekends as well and she couldn't recall the last time she had a well-deserved break either. She was used to having masala chai on an empty stomach, she wasn't having breakfast often because of a lack of time and generally not feeling hungry at all. This is a good sign that she was running on cortisol most of the time which is your stress hormone.

At this point, she was struggling a lot with no idea of what she could do to reduce the symptoms. She really thought she had some sort of serious medical issue going on in her stomach and was even hoping for a diagnosis for it, get it treated with medication and then she would be able to get back to her normal life she had before. She really didn't think that it could have anything to do with her diet or what supplements she was not taking as she had only been taking supplements that she had done before and this had never been a problem. She also thought that because she had managed to improve her health and fitness by changing her diet, she had done all the right things. She would wake up each day and just want to be back to how she was before with no idea what she had to change to get there. Sometimes, you can only go as far as what you know with the tools and resources that you have and you don't know what you don't know. In Gita's case, she was ready to understand more, get the education and take a step further in implementing a different set of tools to feel happier within her own body again.

Gita had already done a stool test before to rule out H pylori, Salmonella, E.coli so me and the team decided that an Organic Acids Test (OATS) would be best to get done at this stage. A urine test is very useful to assess nutritional deficiencies that can affect someone's metabolic pathways. It's a great test to look at the "big picture" of someone's health.

We also got her a blood sugar monitor with testing strips as we suspected that her blood sugars were out of balance. She pricked her finger up to 4 times per day to see how her food impacted her blood sugar levels. It's a useful tool to determine someone's optimal diet and just another great example of how personalized nutrition matters for optimal health in building resiliency.

While Gita's lab tests were sent away to be analysed we got to work straight away on her foundations first as there were a number of cracks we could see that needed healing and correction.

Here's the exact steps we got Gita to take and start implementing:

1. **Having breakfast:** Given the fast paced lifestyle she was living in at the time with her business, breakfast

was missed. So, we got her to start with a small meal to regulate her blood sugars.

2. **Eating more protein:** With each meal which is something a lot of women struggle with for energy and craving control.

3. **Swapping sugary snacks:** For high protein and low sugar options

4. **Hydration:** This was to help reduce the energy crashes and headaches and get her to increase her water intake slowly but surely.

5. **Meal timings:** This was an area that needed a lot of improvement as she was eating whenever she felt like it or whenever she had time due to her busy lifestyle.

6. **Meal prepping:** Sundays was the one day she could catch her breath and get some headspace before a new week started again. We gave her a plan to put in place so that she started her busy week fully supported with foods that were already prepped ahead of time. So, we got her to do some simple batch cooking on a Sunday to avoid her grabbing things last minute, eating unhealthy foods and spending unnecessarily too.

7. **Reducing caffeine:** This is something she relied on like many people to get more energy. Most people start their day in an acidic way which is drinking coffee so we helped her reduce it slowly but surely to allow her body to get used to the changes of energy

boosting foods from her diet and water intake which overall allows the cells to do their work.

So, what did Gita's test results show us? Here's what came up from her OATS test:

1. **Mitochondrial dysfunction:** Mitochondria are the powerhouses of the cell. They help turn the energy we take from food into energy that the cell can use. In Gita's case this was dysfunctional meaning poor energy production.

2. **Methylation issues:** The methylation cycle takes the nutrients from your food and supplements to make the energy your body needs to function properly. Methylation is often referred to as the "B vitamin Cycle" because it uses B vitamins to improve mood, energy, focus, detoxification capabilities, and immune response. In Gita's, she had poor conversion of nutrients into energy.

3. **Digestion:** She also had high levels of Candida, which is a yeast that increases when there is stress, illness, medications such as antibiotics or a high intake of sugary foods. Candida endotoxins can make you feel tired, bloated, trigger headaches and increase intestinal permeability.

4. **Energy:** Her body at the time was not converting fats into energy effectively (fat malabsorption), which was contributing to bloating and gas. To add to this,

she was also not producing enough cellular energy because of a lack of energy-producing cofactors.

5. **Mood:** There was not enough release of Serotonin (the happy chemical) available because of the malabsorption that was present which contributed to mood imbalances

Here are the exact steps we got Gita to take to getting her back to balance with less stress:

Nutrition: We needed to address her nutritional needs first so we started to introduce foods high in B vitamins for energy and methylation like lentils, whole grains, wheat germ, Brazil nuts, peas, spinach, eggs, milk, broccoli, asparagus, mushrooms, almonds, beans, dark leafy greens, oatmeal, buckwheat, dark chocolate. We didn't do all of the things in one go because it can be quite stressful for the body and can also be overwhelming for the mind too and chances of changes succeeding can almost be zero. Gita also struggled with getting some food in her stomach in the morning so we introduced her some milled flaxseed, almonds, brazil nuts, walnuts with CoQ10 to help boost cellular energy. Milled seeds and nuts can be great to add to porridge, greek yoghurt, protein balls and bars (homemade) etc.

Digestion: Due to high levels of Candida we encouraged Gita to introduce more coconut oil, olive oil, garlic, onions and ginger into her diet and how she cooked too. All these foods have antifungal potential. We also got her to avoid any processed sugar, yeast, wine, beer on top of reducing her caffeine intake.

Supplements:

- **Fat digestion and overall digestion:** We got Gita onto Digestive Bitters to help promote healthy digestive processes and give support for a healthy digestive system, promoting digestive enzymes to encourage best absorption of nutrients from the foods she was consuming. She was having 1 dropper as it was in liquid form before each meal. She continued this throughout the whole journey.
- **Probiotics for Candida:** Saccharomyces Boulardii can inhibit populations of Candida and prevent them from establishing in the intestines. Gita was taking 1 to 2 capsules per day.
- **Energy:** We got her some B-complex vitamins on 1 capsule every other day in the morning or afternoon gradually moving it onto 1 capsule every day.
- **Peppermint:** To reduce the bloating and gas she was experiencing.
- **Boswellia:** Boswellia Serata is actually a tree native to India, Africa and the Arabian Peninsula and also goes by the name of Indian Frankincense. Boswellia

helps to reduce inflammation due to the active compounds found to be anti-inflammatory.

So, what were Gita's results after 12 weeks and implementing a lot of changes? Below are the true results she received from her hard work of making solid changes:

- Her symptoms reduced by 85%
- Barely no tea/coffee in the last 4-6 weeks
- Bloating and gas were almost completely gone
- Cramps disappeared
- Sleep was much better with still the odd night or two of waking up in the middle of the night
- Energy was better than where she was before however more changes needed to be made within her own time management as well.
- No more Quorn which is a meat substitute made out of by fermenting Fusarium venenatum, a natural fungus found in soil.
- Snacking on Nairn's instead of sugary biscuits/chocolate
- Good breakfasts were implemented which consisted of eggs, mushrooms. pancakes, yogurt with linseeds.
- Tesco online shopping to work smarter with her time and not harder
- Her blood sugars improved as well

We worked with Gita two years ago and since catching up with her recently for my book, I asked her how she was really doing after 2 years. I was eager to find out if she had kept up with the changes and stuck to them. In her own words, this is was she had to say:

"I continued with the pre / probiotics for a while but have stopped since. I have reduced my sugar intake and continued to eat more protein and less processed foods. I have continued to indulge on Nairn's biscuits instead of other snacks whenever possible but allowed myself to have some of my favourite desserts when I really wanted them. Thank you so much for all your help. I am so much different to what I was before I started my work with you".

Chapter 3
World War 3

One of my favourite musical artists of all time is Nerina Pallot and she wrote a song called 'Everybody's Gone To War' which actually sparked the inspiration for this chapter of the book. I'd like to rephrase the song title to 'Every Body Has Gone To War' for the purpose of this chapter. If you haven't heard of this song, I'd highly recommend that you go and listen to it and let me know what you think of it.

I don't believe that Covid was a health crisis / war which may trigger you slightly as you read it but stay with me. I do believe however, what Covid did was really show and shed light on the unhealthy war that is happening right now inside out in each and every one of us and we are completely blind to it.

Have you ever questioned why in such a modern digital world you live in with access to incredible facts, figures, knowledge, materials and experts yet the population are the sickest we have ever been?

Obesity at an all-time high, depression rates going up and up, an individual losing someone close to them to suicide, everyone seems to be suffering with anxiety, IBS8 and has been diagnosed and labelled with ADHD.

Makes you wonder right?

It's my belief that as human beings, we are constantly going to war every day. What I mean by this is imagine waking up every day and going out to war, like physically? And if you can't imagine that, then imagine this that is happening inside your body 24/7. The amount of inflammation that's building up all of the time, the amount of disconnect, the amount of unfulfillment that's happening inside of so many people right now. I call this an inside job because it's literally what it is.

What Is Inflammation?

There's two sides to inflammation you need to understand when it comes to building resilience with your immune system and overall improving gut function and they are acute and chronic inflammation.

Acute inflammation is basically inflammation that is sudden, intense, painful and lasts for a short period of time such as a tissue injury like a cut, infections etc.

Chronic inflammation is inflammation that is consistently there and sticks around for a lot longer and in some cases a lifetime. Examples of chronic inflammation are IBS, arthritis, fibromyalgia, constipation etc.

How Does Inflammation Work On A Biochemical Level?

The best way to explain and remember how inflammation works is through playing Cops and Robbers.

It'll be fun, I promise ;)

Think of inflammation as the superhero of your body because when there is a sign of trouble, inflammation rushes in to rescue and protect you and of course, save the day.

The Robbers: Inflammatory Triggers

The reason why inflammation starts in the first place is because of inflammatory triggers such as cuts, scrapes, bacteria, viruses etc. Your body detects this like a house alarm going off when an intruder is present in a home and sends off an alarm.

The Emergency Call Center: Cytokines

Cytokines are basically small proteins that allow your cells to talk to each other and they play a huge role in regulating your immune system. Cytokines are the emergency police headquarters of your body. If Cytokines could speak, they would be shouting out, "We've got a situation here!"

The Cops: The White Blood Cells

White blood cells are another set of superheroes of your immune system. If they had a torch then they are looking for any signs of trouble by consistently checking the body out. When they get the call from cytokines, they rush to the scene. They're like the cops trying to restore order and calm the situation down.

The Backup: The Inflammatory Mediators

Now that the white blood cells have arrived at the scene and seen what a mess the inflammatory triggers have made, they realise very quickly that they are going to need back up. The inflammatory mediators are the weapons of mass peace that your body uses to fight the robbers aka inflammatory triggers. These include things like prostaglandins and leukotrienes. Pretty cool and complex names for a weapon right? I can just hear it now when a police officer says, "hang on let me load up my Leukotrienes" haha! They help white blood cells attack the robbers and repair any damage.

The Forensics Team: Macrophages

After the battle, your body needs a forensics team to go through the mess and clean it all up. Macrophages are like the cleaners of your immune system. They clean up the mess left behind by the fight and help with healing.

Inflammation is a crucial part for healing however it's not meant to go on forever. Your body has a built-in "off" switch. Once the threat is gone, anti-inflammatory molecules step in to calm things down. This prevents inflammation from getting out of control and keeps inflammation at a good balance.

Chronic inflammation is where things start to go wrong for the long term and your superhero system keeps attacking even when there's no real threat to the body at the time. Why this happens isn't very clear however it is my belief that when you consistently don't have a well-rounded diet that works for you, not getting enough sleep, drinking too much alcohol, not managing your stress levels or not even aware how stressed you really are, have negatives thoughts that go round and round possibly resulting in overwhelm, anxiety, imposter syndrome, not feeling good enough can cause too much inflammation for the body to deal with at any given time. It becomes an overload release of cortisol for the body to start sorting out and getting it back to balance.

Chapter 4
The Gut

Most people think that digestion starts when you take your first bite, however it actually starts in the mind also known as the Cephalic Phase and this is where you start to smell, hear and see about foods and your mouth starts to build up with saliva.

The food enters your mouth where enzymes start breaking down the carbohydrates and while your teeth start the mechanical chewing part of the process. The food then is passed down the oesophagus and enters the stomach. The stomach is where the gastric juices of Hydrochloric (HCL) acid breaks it down. HCL acts as a disinfectant and often leans on the Liver & Gallbladder to add more juice to break it down. It then enters the small & large intestine where absorption happens, vital nutrients are taken from the food to fuel cells and then excreted.

Here's a really important thing I want you to take away from understanding the Gut is…

You are not what you eat…

You are what you absorb, digest and excrete. If you and

I ate the exact same plate of food, the results of how much of that plate of food is absorbed by your body, digested and excreted would be two totally different results.

What Does The Gut Do For Us?

It's known as the Second Brain and it doesn't need permission from the brain to do its work, it acts as its "own brain". There are more than 100 Million brain cells in the Gut which tells you that it's very powerful in thinking for itself. It has more neurons than the spinal cord and the peripheral nervous system.

The Enteric Nervous System (ENS) which controls the digestion and elimination part and works by itself is a huge part of the Peripheral Nervous System (PNS) that can control gastrointestinal behaviour. You may also be familiar with the mind and body connection and this is to do with the Vagus Nerve. This carries 90% of information in the fibres from the gut to the brain. The brain interprets gut signals as emotions so anytime you ever felt like you need to trust your gut instincts or you've had that gut feeling then make no mistake that this is true information fed to you via the vagus nerve.

Have you ever had those days where you have feelings

of happiness when eating food and it just puts you in a good mood? Well, 95% of Serotonin is in The Gut. Serotonin is known as the happy chemical and 95% of this neurotransmitter is in The Gut. Food does affect your mood and when you are eating fats and carbohydrates, this tends to increase the feelings of happiness and pleasure which not increases Serotonin but Dopamine too which is another chemical like Serotonin.

So many people in the UK are always fighting off colds and flus because it's that "time of the year" to catch one. However, 75% of your immune system is in The Gut which tells you that if you have a good functioning gut then the chances of you having a heavy cold or flu is a lot slimmer and recovering from one would be a lot quicker too.

So, what can you do for your Gut?

Your food choices have a huge impact on the composition and diversity of your gut microbiota. Generally having a diet that is quite rich in fiber, which is found in fruits, vegetables, whole grains, and legumes, is like a massive feast for your microorganisms. The fiber that you eat helps the growth of beneficial bacteria.

On the other hand, if your diet is high in processed foods, sugar, and saturated fats then this can change the gut microbiomes in many ways that are damaging to your health. It can lead to an overgrowth of harmful bacteria and a decrease in beneficial ones, potentially contributing to various health issues, including weight gain, inflammation, and even mental health disorders.

This is why it's so important to understand that your nutrition and your relationship with the foods that you eat are unique and have to be personalized, not download a diet plan off Google or something generic. Google doesn't take into account your biochemistry or your Psychology other than monitoring your behaviour online.

Here are some typical signs of a dysfunctional gut:

- Poor quality of sleep so waking up in the middle of the night
- Bloating
- Gas
- Skin issues/outbreaks
- Weight gain/weight loss
- Feeling tired all the time
- Hair thinning
- Achy joints & muscles
- Low mood

- Low energy
- Negative thinking more than usual
- Diarrhoea
- Constipation
- Acid reflux
- Crohn's Disease
- Ulcerative Colitis

So, what causes The Gut to become dysfunctional?

High Stress: Having high stress levels where it's not been managed well leads to fight, flight or freeze response. This is also where less blood & nutrient flow to the digestive system, signal failures towards the pancreas, liver, gall bladder to release juices is less so food isn't broken down properly. Examples of common everyday stress would be work related stress with financial worries, zero hour contracts, deadlines, travel, long hours, no/little movement due to desk based jobs. It can be family stress with looking after bills, the family and bringing up children as well as looking after loved ones.

Poor food choices: If you are not taking the time to be more present with food and chewing it enough, having distractions at meal times, eating while working and eating in places where you would feel stressed can cause dysfunction to the Gut over time.

Prescribed medications and poor quality of supplements: This can disrupt the gut bacteria and can even wipe out good bacteria at the same time.

Poor Posture: Having a more slouched posture can add more physical strain to the back, the spine and your stomach which can often misdirect stomach acid into the wrong direction.

Environment: Your environment absolutely shapes so where you live, the relationships you (personal/professional), the air that you breathe play a massive part on how your body receives and manages stress.

Trauma: Having gone through past hurts, conflicts, grievances, bereavement, loss can cause trauma to the nervous system therefore experiencing fight, flight, freeze all of the time.

In this book, I am going to be sharing with you strategies and tips that will help you as you go deeper into expanding your knowledge into Gut dysfunctionalities and the foundations of your health in the next chapter.

Testing For Gut Issues

The problem I see and hear time and time again is that society will just go on some crazy diet of eating nothing or sold on a sugary shake or a pill/supplement to get rid of the problem. Your gut system is delicate and intelligent and unfortunately does not respond well to a quick fix approach.

An estimated 13 million people in the UK alone have IBS issues yet it seems to be on the rise and more and more people are just getting sicker and sicker as a result of a weakened immune system. I mean, go figure!

So, my best advice for you would be to always start with the foundations that you will read about in Chapter 5 and then look into getting your gut tested. You will understand some of the functional tests I've gotten my clients to do in this book and the reasons behind it and what the data truly led me and the team down to helping that individual overcome their health challenges.

Look At Your Own Shit

In the meantime, I want to point you in the right direction of some tools and resources you can start using in getting an insight into your gut health.

If you are ever concerned or just generally curious to what your poop is really telling you, then start to actually take notice of what times of the day you empty your bowel, what's the color of your poo, what's the consistency and how long you were sitting on the toilet seat for. All this information before you even go down the route of testing can help you to help your body out so much more. The only time Google has its good uses for information is searching for the Bristol Stool Chart. It was developed in 1997 at the University of Bristol to classify poop into seven different types and give a quick overview on what the body may be telling you.

Type 1: Tends to be separate hard lumps which can be quite difficult to excrete out with almost like a push/strain like behaviour. This can often indicate that you are constipated and that your body has taken water from you in order to carry out digestion and other functions. Often in a constipated state, dehydration is usually the culprit so make sure you address your water intake and get plenty of it into self-correct constipation.

Type 2: Is normally lumpy and sausage like and can indicate that you may be slightly constipated. Follow the guidelines from type 1 to self-correct type 2 poop.

Type 3: Comes in like a sausage shape with some cracks in it and this is basically normal.

Type 4: Is the opposite in terms of shape from type 3 because Type 4 is like a smooth, soft sausage type of shape that is also normal.

Type 5: Is very different from the other types and can often come in as soft blobs with clear edges and that can indicate that you may be lacking some fiber so if you ever experience this then definitely look at your diet and see where more fiber can be added so self-correct this type back to type 3 and 4.

Type 6: This is where your poop comes out in a very mushy consistency with the edges being ragged. This can indicate inflammation is present where stool testing can come in very useful to find out more.

Type 7: This is where your poop is just liquid form and holds no shape or consistency whatsoever. This indicates inflammation and diarrhea is present. As previously mentioned, stool testing can come in very useful to find out more.

Now, you may experience type 1, 2, 5, 6, 7 once a week or once in a while or just a one off. If it's a one off then you can easily address it by simply looking at hydration, movement, the foods that you eat and how much you are moving around day to day. Monitor how your body responds and then see if your poop goes back to being more like type 3 and 4. However, if you are experiencing constipation, watery poop, diarrhoea then chances are that something else is causing the inflammation in your gut and as a result it's not coming out as type 3 and 4.

Don't Be A Supplement Whore

Supplements are usually the last thing I get clients onto when sorting their gut health issues out because no supplement is going to work if your gut lining is damaged through stress and inflammation. It'll just get passed through your body and out through urine and waste. You end up with just really expensive pee. The body's ability to absorb as much as it needs to is a lot less when it's inflamed inside and when the gut is compromised.

Through my experience and years of being in the health and wellness industries, I have developed a bullshit scam detector to spot the scam when it comes to health.

Here they are:

1. Health experts telling you that their supplements are the best on the planet and that there is nothing else

like it on the market right now! Bullshit Detector Results: 10/10

2. So called "Health Experts" emerging from the Multilevel marketing businesses letting you know that their golden morning shake has everything in it to set you up for the day. Please, most of them have nothing but sugar helping you to get to Diabetes a lot quicker. Bullshit Detector Results: 10/10

3. Chucking a diagnosis or a strategy in your face for you to get on without properly explaining the why and expecting you to just get on with it. Health isn't and shouldn't be guess work and it's about looking at an individual as a whole and not a symptom. Bullshit Detector Results: 10/10

4. Those "health experts" telling you that their "thing" (whatever this thing is) works for everyone. No it doesn't and is a complete lie because they have failed to realise and understand that every single human being on this planet is incredibly unique and original. Bullshit Detector Results: 10/10

But nothing pisses me off more when health experts promote shit supplements and abuse people's emotions in getting them to buy them so that they can make money or move up a level in their business.

I don't have anything against MLM businesses, it's the person promoting and driving a dangerous message that worries me because their intentions are not in the best interest of the person in need.

Becoming a health expert many years ago, required me to show up and walk the talk and to show a level of vulnerability. It also meant taking ownership, being responsible for my own results as well as the fact that the advice that I gave people was truly going to help them.

Something my good friend Greg has always said to me and his clients:

"Would you trust a personal trainer with your hair and nails? If not, why would you trust a beautician with your nutrition"?

Makes you think, doesn't it?

Chapter 5

Gut Health And Stress

Imagine how a house is built. You would never start building the roof of the house first without building the floor plan first otherwise the roof would collapse.

I want you to take this same approach with your health. You have to understand your own foundations to your own health first before you go down the root of spending lots of time, energy and money into anything and everything just to get rid of the pain that you may be in.

I see it time and time again, an individual in pain who's been fed bullshit that a supplement would cure their problem, or going on a 21 day cleanse will get rid of the crap that the body needs to get rid of or painkillers that will just diminish the pain forever and all is right again. Or better yet, had a colonoscopy done and it's all come back normal so nothing is wrong.

Let's just say, you have had experience with some of these approaches and the pain never came back again in your mind. I'm sorry to burst your bubble, because if you haven't fully understood the root of why that pain has occurred, all you have done is delayed or redirected that issue to another place in the body or changed the date of when that pain reappears again with a vengeance.

The foundations of your health is absolutely crucial to how you function everyday, how you show up for yourself and others and how you survive and thrive while living on this earth.

In this chapter, I am going to take you through my entire Stressed To Success system so that you come away with a solid understanding of what it is you need to do always before going down the quick fix route which over time will cost you a lot more and I am not just talking about money alone. I'm also going to talk in depth of how each foundation is connected to the gut and how it is affected.

I want to start talking about stress first and foremost because it's stress that contributes to dis-eases, illness, pain and it's what starts the beautiful journey of pain.

The word 'Stress' has been abused, stretched and is often spoken in a way of how so many people talk about the weather to fit people's comfort levels. However, the more you use and understand it loosely, and don't acknowledge and understand why you are experiencing a particular level of stress; you miss the signs and clues your body gives you to turn a corner and change it around. There are physical, emotional and mental stresses that occur every day and it tends to show up as weight gain, lack of motivation to get things done in business, not stepping up and taking the lead (not because we want to), forgetfulness, overwhelm, and generally feeling doubtful and overthinking.

In a nutshell, stress is a feeling of emotional or physical tension. It can come from any event or thought that makes you feel frustrated, angry, or nervous. Stress is your body's reaction to a challenge or demand. In short bursts, stress can be positive, such as when it helps you avoid danger or meet a deadline.

Stress is also known as the steroid hormone called Cortisol. Cortisol controls a wide range of crucial processes throughout the body, including your metabolism and the immune response and of course, you need cortisol to survive too. So, I don't want you to think that stress is a bad thing, it only becomes an issue when you don't know what type of stress or stresses are triggering the pain as well as how long you've had it for. The more chronic your stress levels become, the more problems tend to occur everywhere in the body.

Stress is like a switch, the longer the stress switch is on, the more cortisol is released into the body continuously, causing all sorts of mayhem and signal failures and all the systems in the body work tirelessly 24/7 to create equilibrium and harmony in the body. It's basically fighting for you, putting out all the fires as much as it can so that you function and stay alive every single day.

The moment you feel pain or a symptom has shown up in your body, please note that you have taken your body too far. The worse thing is, most people ignore this part or pop some pills to make it all go away and carry on as normal. Your body is very intelligent and you can't outrun it so most people will end up being forced to stay in bed, pop pills and just 'live' with it so please note at this stage, your body is seriously crying out for help.

Stress affects every system in your body such as the Musculoskeletal system, Respiratory System, Cardiovascular System, Endocrine System, Hormone Production, Immune System, Digestive System, Reproductive System, Nervous System and so on.

Now, I am not telling you all this to scare you but more to create awareness because once you are aware, you can do something about it, something better for the long term so that you don't run into a dis-eased state and complications arise.

Chapter 6

Gut Health And Sugar

Sugar is a natural ingredient that has always been part of the human diet. Some sugars are found naturally in foods (e.g. fruit, vegetables and milk) while others are used during processing and cooking. Carbohydrates composed of sugars and starches are broken down in your body into glucose. Sugars are an important source of energy with glucose being the most important for your body. You need sugar to function properly, which is mainly glucose as an example, your brain requires around 130 grams of glucose per day to keep functioning so it's not all bad. However, the harmful sugars are commonly found in processed foods (think cake, biscuits, carbonated soft drinks), as well as highly concentrated natural sources such as fruit juice and honey.

Your body does not distinguish between sugars used in food and drink that is manufactured or in the home, and those found naturally in fruits and vegetables. For example, the sucrose in an apple is broken down in exactly the same way as the sucrose in your sugar bowl. However, the rate of which sucrose is absorbed can vary depending on if the source is a solid or liquid food, for example in an apple or apple juice.

I do feel sugars and carbs get a bad reputation for being the 'devil' when it comes to health and I do understand that sugar is almost in everything. However, the responsibility falls on the user meaning you. It's your responsibility to do your research on what nutritional value the foods and drinks you consume have. Every year, there's always going to be a brand new supplement, food and/or drink that's been labelled as 'healthy' go onto the supermarket shelves and people rush and spend their money on it, kidding themselves that they are eating healthy. It makes me laugh and frustrated at the same time when I see high protein breads in the supermarket classed as 'high protein' just because they've sprinkled seeds on top of it; or low fat yogurts classed as 'healthy' but when you look at the carbohydrate amount in that one yogurt pot, it's just high in sugar with no fat in it, or 'healthy' fruit smoothies in the morning.

If something is marketed as 'healthy', it will sell with no emotional attachment to whether it's really healthy or not to the consumer. It's marketing 101 where a business needs to market the product to sell to the masses and say exactly what the consumer wants on the packaging. As long as it sells and makes somebody a lot of money, it's all good and does the job (said with a sarcastic tone). The Health Food Industry in the UK alone is worth over £3 billion[1]. All I am saying is, it's not going to stop because your needs change, different health problems arise every year and there are going to be many companies out there that will bring out organic healthy food and drinks literally to the table. There will be some that are really good and some that don't quite cut it. Just do your research for your own good.

Always look at the sugars at the back of all your products to see exactly just how much there actually is in one product. It's usually right after carbohydrates and right underneath it would say, 'of which sugars'.

It's all well and good understanding what's out there when you go shopping but I want to educate you on why the body can only handle a small amount of sugar and what actually happens when you over consume sugar in one day and how it starts messing up your gut. This way you have both the inside and outside perspective of the sweet stuff.

A healthy gut is built around balance! Sugar is mostly absorbed into your body through your small intestine. Your small intestine can only process a certain amount of sugar. Many studies have shown that if you eat the equivalent of roughly 25 g - 30 g of sugar in one go (approximately seven teaspoons), the small intestine can't process all of that sugar meaning some travels down into the large intestine and eventually into the liver through the bloodstream2. For context, a single can of Coke is already over this seven teaspoon threshold – so, it's really not huge amounts to mess with your gut.

When the cells in your gut are exposed to a lot of sugar all of the time, this is where poor health starts and where your immune system unfortunately is compromised.

Bottom line is the less sugar that the small intestine needs to process, the less hard work the large intestine will need to do as well as your liver, bloods etc.

The Dopamine Reward System

The Dopamine Reward System gets activated when we eat sweet foods. Dopamine is a brain chemical released by neurons and can signal that an event was positive. When the reward system fires, it reinforces behaviours making it more likely for you to carry out these actions again3. Unfortunately, our brains are still functionally very similar to our ancestors, and it really likes sugar. When the reward system has been repeatedly activated by stimulants like drugs, alcohol, sex, shopping, exercise, foods etc, it causes the brain to adapt to frequent stimulation, leading to a sort of tolerance.

Question for you to think about right now… How many times in the day or your week do you feel stimulated from the foods you eat?

And when you don't, what do you replace it with to feel content?

We need stimulation but we tend to go for the wrong things to get stimulated from consistently.

A Pint Of Sugar Anyone?

I was so blind to my sugar intake years ago and just how stressed out I was and how much I relied on food and drink to make me feel good in the moment.

Exactly 5 months after my father passed away, I became very good at hiding my pain behind my smiles. For most of 2018, I felt quite numb and I didn't really do much about my health even though I was feeling pain in my joints and muscles but the worst of it all was in my stomach. I just ignored it all, wishfully thinking everything is going to be ok. I would look at myself in the mirror and just feel shame and disgust at how much I let go of my body compared to how I used to look. I used to feel proud of myself but I just felt disappointment, I didn't feel in control anymore. I started to cope by having really long naps, take outs because I had no motivation to cook, eating more chocolate and doughnuts than usual. It was this huge black void and I just ended up just filling it with unhealthy habits mainly sugary foods because it was cheap, quick and easy to find comfort for a little while. That was my way of coping - burying my head in the sand and I did it for ages. It got to a point that the intense burning I had in my stomach was just too painful. I was literally cowered over my bed in pain. I could no longer sleep anymore which left me feeling tired, unfocused and burnout most of the time. Enough was enough and I was sick and tired of feeling like shit all of the time.

It was time to stop ignoring what my body was telling me for so long and start listening to it and looking after it in the right way. To cut down and slow down.

The easiest thing I could start looking at was my diet before getting into the deep stuff.

Here is what a typical diet looked like for me and I am going to show how much sugar I consumed in a day, particularly when I used to label it a stressful day.

Breakfast - a bowl of porridge (16.2g with 8 g of sugar, honey - 10G) with milk washed down with a cup of coffee with 2 sugars(16g) banana - 27.2 g

= 78 g

Snack - natural bars (15.6g) and crisps (1.1g)

= 17g

Lunch - sandwich,(3.6g) sprite,(11g) chocolate bar, (44.7g) pineapple fruit,(16.6) crisps(1.1g)

= 77g

Snack - crisps and coffee with 2 sugars milk

= 17g

Coffee:

16g

2 beers, (1g) bottle of wine(58g)

= 60g

Dinner - takeout pizza (5 slices - 25g)

= 25g

Stay up late and watch Netflix and eat more crisps, (2.2g) chocolate junk food! (44.7)

= 52g

TOTAL: 350g

If you add up the entire day's worth of sugar, it would be a pint. If someone handed you a pint of sugar, would you eat it? I hope you are shaking your head with a firm no. But the reality was this is what I was doing as my stressful days were not managed well, my emotional and mental world were chaotic until I crashed and burned. I thought porridge, banana, Tesco's Chicken salad sandwich and getting some fruit into my diet was healthy but when you look at overall, it's really not when you do it too much.

These 'stressful' days went on for ages. I was really slow and sluggish at just getting started in the morning. I struggled to just fully be present with my early morning clients and heavily relied on coffee to just get started. I needed more and more naps in the afternoon like 3 to 4 hours because I would literally crash on my living room sofa. I wasn't able to get a lot done on my to-do list either so this added to my frustration and I constantly shamed and judged myself for being 'lazy'.

I had difficulty remembering things and my focus and my attention was just blurred so which means I probably lost out on many opportunities that were right under my nose to grow and scale my business at the time and to develop myself personally too. The one that hurt the most was that it hit my finances! I was the problem! I also totally put any romantic relationships/interests on the back burner because I had put on weight that I was just not proud of and I didn't like the way my clothes just didn't fit me anymore. My breasts grew an unhealthy size and started to get a bit of a wobbly tummy which led me to just hide behind baggier clothes and knocked my confidence out of the park in just feeling good in my own skin! And getting those unhelpful comments from family members does not help at all either where they look at you up and down and come up to your face and ask, 'you've put on a bit'? It used to wind me up so much that I would be thinking about that comment for days and have a good cry.

Body shaming is not cool and never will be. You have no idea what the person might be going through and how hurtful a comment can be to that person so always be kind and compassionate towards others and yourself.

Chapter 7
Gut Health And Sleep

My sleep was horrendous back when I created and ran my very first business back in 2012. I had the attitude of 'Work Hard, Play Harder', be part of the '5am Club' or 'I'll Sleep When I'm dead' or I used to think naively that I could 'catch up' on sleep at the weekend. This is not how sleep works and certainly not how the body functions to get the rest it needs.

I used to work on and off my business 7 days a week and I still factored in partying, drinking, eating crap foods, working out (the one that I did the most), family and friends (the one that I did least) and I just didn't get enough sleep in. I could run on very little sleep, work all day and then crash by 6pm in the evening in complete exhaustion. The more I lived this type of lifestyle, the more I messed up the natural rhythm of my body which is known as the Circadian Rhythm.

The Circadian Rhythm

The more I started to learn about my natural body clock, the more it started to make sense to me about alertness, focus, productivity, calming my nervous system down to rest and digest and the best way to achieve it. I realised how much I was damaging the natural system I already had which did this amazing job of getting the rest that I needed and helping me function everyday. If there one thing that started to give me the biggest wins in health and in my business was getting sleep right for my body.

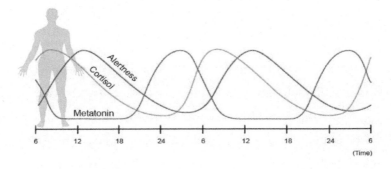

Using this book as inspiration, make a promise to yourself to really make the effort to understand the above diagram well and how it works. When you achieve that, you are onto the right track in getting the right amount of energy into your day, every day.

It's a 24 hour internal clock that is running the night and day patterns in the background of your entire body. It's more powerful than any other clock out there. So, where is this clock located? It's located in the hypothalamus, which is inside of your brain and its job is to coordinate your autonomic nervous system. It controls your body temperature, it sends signals to let you know when you are thirsty and hungry.

Turn your attention to the bottom of the diagram where 24 hour times are shown and start with 6. The squiggly lines show:

Melatonin: Sleep Hormone
Cortisol: Stress Hormone
Alertness

Melatonin as you can see from the diagram is low during the day and then peaks towards the early start of the evening. This is to prepare you for sleep when it's high and allow cortisol to wake you up and feel more alert when it's low.

Cortisol is needed in your body for survival and alertness. At 6am in the morning, your cortisol hormone is at its highest so it releases around about six o'clock in the morning and rightly because this is when most people tend to get up to go to work.
You can see just after 6pm in the evening, Melatonin actually does this crossover with Cortisol where it starts

to reduce down to about 3pm/4pm in the afternoon. Afternoon dips can actually be quite normal because your stress hormone is going down allowing you to unwind and get ready to go to sleep. Melatonin is at its highest after midnight, so between 1am to 3am,you can actually achieve deep sleep and get good rest. So, this is what a normal functioning sleep pattern actually looks like. There's many ups and downs and that both hormones release more or less at different times for a specific reason, and this cycle is literally repeated every 24 hours.

Dysfunctional sleep patterns tend to take shape when you are still switched on and working away into the evening when Melatonin needs to be released. Instead, Cortisol is still hanging around a lot longer so that it helps you stay more alert to finish the activity or task at hand.

Many people are still working away on their laptops, on their iPads and phones and on Zoom calls and just constantly switched on. Many people will tend to rely on a lot of sugary drinks and foods, caffeine to just get them through the day. So, the more you are working away, the more you're exposed to unnatural light from your screens and laptops and digital devices, the more melatonin can't do its job and release itself and have that restful period that you need throughout the night. This is why deep rested sleep becomes shorter and shorter and why so many people tend to wake up feeling tired and wired at the same time. Your 24 cycle doesn't stop, it will keep going but in a dysfunctional way if you don't put in place a stop button of some sort. Health issues start to happen when you don't actually sort your sleep patterns and make it a priority.

You are designed to have a 24 hour rhythm in your physiology and your metabolism. It's an absolute pattern that you must stick to get you fully functioning as a human being. Sleep is fundamental because it determines when to eat too so your sleep patterns have to be correct in order for your body to do its job when it comes to processing food with very little distractions.

If you are a parent with young children then work on your sleep patterns day by day till you get into a good rhythm that matches the 24 hour sleep pattern. If you are someone that does a lot of night shifts and is awake when most people are asleep then definitely incorporate more stress relieving strategies like walks, deep breathing, meditation into your days off to help reduce the stress of working against the 24 hour sleep pattern.

How Sleep Actually Works

Each stage of sleep has a very distinctive, restorative quality style, a different type of resting. Through different stages of sleep and how you move through each phase plays a really big important role in your health and over the course of the next few days after. You go through several 90 minute cycles and each cycle plays a really important role in maintaining your mental and physical health. Your sleep is divided into two categories: non rapid eye movement (NRE) and rapid eye movement (REM). REM means where your eye tends to move really, really quickly, almost like a flutter under the eyelid. It's these two types of sleep cycles that make up a single cycle. Your brain progresses sequentially as it goes in a sequence through each stage of sleep.

Wake Cycle: The amount of time you are awake when you are in bed before and after falling asleep. So, when your head hits the pillow, do you tend to fall asleep quickly or toss and turn for a bit? Part of the Wake Cycle is also moments where you wake up for 5 to 10 seconds and then go back to sleep again.

Light Sleep: This cycle initiates your sleep cycle and as a transition. You have to go through this stage in order to get to Deep sleep and REM stage. Muscles start to become more relaxed, your heart rate and your breathing tends to slow down however you can end up waking up quite easily. It just means you are not in a deep sleep state yet.

Deep Sleep: In this part of the sleep cycle, your breathing slows down, your heart rate decreases, and your body temperature drops so this is where the deep sleep starts to begin. Deep sleep is where you can reap the benefits of recovery and rejuvenation. What I mean is this is where your body focuses on muscle growth and repair as well as the waste removal in your brain. It would be difficult to wake up in a deep sleep state. If you ever woken up unexpectedly, you would wake up feeling groggy and disoriented.

REM: Rapid eye movement is essential to just re-energizing your mind. It's associated with dreaming, with memory, learning and problem solving. It's also where you can experience vivid dreams and your body's clever too because in this stage it keeps you still so you don't end up acting out your dreams.

So, your body goes through these cycles four or five times each night. Some of the cycles tend to start earlier in the night to have more non rapid eye movement sleep rather than later. However, by the final cycle, when you go into a rapid eye movement, your body may even sort of tend to just skip the non-rapid eye movement entirely. The key point here is being mindful of caffeine and sugar intake, alcohol intake, and your intake of foods. All of these things affect your sleep and how long you get to spend in each of the cycles.

If you really want to understand your sleep patterns more, there are some good apps that can help you track it better, Fitbits and Oura rings definitely can give you more depth to your sleep patterns too.

How Does Gut Health Affect The Quality Of Sleep

There are many reasons why you may not be able to get a good night's sleep. It could be physical stress such as an injury, you could also be overthinking about things, having a late dinner, watching TV till late or drinking a lot of caffeine/alcoholic drinks in the day.

Some of these reasons may be obvious and sometimes you can bring our sleep back to balance and have a good night's sleep. However, what is becoming more and more apparent is your Digestive Health, in particular is how your gut bacteria behaves in your digestive tract.

The following factors can affect the gut to become dysfunctional:

High stress: If you are not managing your stress properly, your body is in constant fight, flight or freeze mode allowing very little opportunity to rest and recover at night.

Poor diet: If your diets are takeaways the majority of the time, processed foods, high in sugar then this will definitely suppress your sleep hormone known as Melatonin.

Heavy meals: If your meal timings and quantity is off and more than usual, this puts the digestive system under more pressure to process the foods meaning it has to work over time to get the job done. This results in poor sleep.

Just high stress levels and a poor diet alone can cause you to feel overwhelmed, lack focus and concentration, anxiety and overthinking. All of these emotions can fester and keep you awake at night.

There has been many studies and research in the last 5 years giving us an insight into how gut bacteria can affect your circadian rhythm. Gut bacteria are microorganisms that live in the digestive tract of humans. They play important roles in the body including communicating with other systems, breaking down and utilising fats, proteins and carbohydrates as well as producing certain vitamins.

Therefore, it's no surprise that a lack of sleep and appetite impacts how our gut bacteria behave. Our gut bacteria need diversity meaning it needs a range of good quality foods consistently to have a good supply of good bacteria in our digestive tract. If we are sleep deprived, this can decrease our appetite leading us to crave more processed, sugary foods which can impact the diversity of our gut bacteria.

How Can You Start To Improve Your Sleep Quality?

I'm not going to use this space and tell you that you need pillows packed with duck feathers or a mattress that has memory foam built into it and has a double layer of extra sponge that helps you sleep better. I am sure it does contribute to the quality of your sleep and you can go and research this in your own time as part of your sleep regime.

However, keeping in line with the theme of this book, I'm going to get straight to the point on what really helps improve the quality of your sleep.

First and foremost, you must adopt a better diet consisting of more green leafy, cruciferous vegetables, using good quality fats like coconut oil on high heat and olive oil for salad and marinades. You should also consider better quality lean meats and proteins and good sources of carbohydrates too. As you know by now, food and sugar makes a huge impact with your gut so this section shouldn't all be that surprising when it comes to achieving a good quality sleep.

Your bedroom should be in complete darkness at bedtime so that you can get the much needed rest and a better chance of going through the different stages of sleep to achieve good recovery and strengthen your immune system[7].

Avoid blue light exposure in the evenings and in your bedroom. Studies have shown that the timing of light exposure plays a huge role in your circadian rhythm. The more you expose different types of lights at night time, it can block melatonin to increase when it needs to help you sleep. Therefore, the timing of light exposure is very important from when you wake up to when you retire for the evening[4]. Mobile phones and laptops and other electronic devices are kryptonite for your sleep in the evening time so when you can agree to switch at a certain time, stick to it.

Chapter 8
Gut Health And Hydration

In my expert opinion, hydration means way more than just drinking eight glasses of water a day. It is also about taking responsibility to understand it at a cellular level too5. Why? Because your cells need hydration to maintain their structure and function and for your body to function on a day to day basis too.

You lose water in four different ways which are through:

1. Urine
2. Sweating
3. Breathing
4. Poop

Your body is made up for more than 70% water and your kidneys are the organs to monitor how much water your body has had.

Your brain and kidneys contains around 83% water

Your lungs contain around 85%

Your blood contain around 94%

Your eyes contain around 95%

Your heart contains up to 75% and your muscles contain around 80%.

So, you can see that hydration goes above and beyond just looking at how yellow your urine is, in fact your whole being needs good quality hydration to function optimally and for you to stay focused.

To understand hydration and life, you need to understand cells and how they work.

Your cells are the first sign of life because it comes from a molecule to an atom and creates your organs to then create you.

Fascinating right?

Cells provide structure for the body as it takes in nutrients from foods. It converts these nutrients into energy, and carries out specific functions that you need to carry out. Without water, your cells can't move any waste and byproducts that your body obviously produces. It also can't take in any nutrients that you take from the foods that you eat. It can't transport from cell to cell, it just basically can't function and it can't signal to other cells to do other jobs. So, there's a massive breakdown in communication when your cells do not get the right amount of hydration. To open your eyes more, there's more than 37. 2 trillion cells in the human body. That's a humongous amount of cells per person.

All of those trillions of cells need an adequate amount of water every single day to function really, really well otherwise you lose your focus and energy.

How To Hydrate Properly

Now that you know you have more than 37 trillion cells in your body bouncing off one another, I want to take you another layer deeper into hydration.

Every single cell in your body right now has batteries and they are called Mitochondria. It's what gives you energy every single day. It's the mitochondria in the cells that use the hydrogen in water to make energy which is also known as Adenosine Triphosphate (ATP). This takes me back to the science lessons back in the school days.

There are hydro molecules in water which makes the energy and it's also the hydrogen molecules that bind to free radicals and get rid of inflammation. Hydration is also what keeps inflammation really, really low in your body as well. Every day your body deals with all sorts of inflammation from free radicals from stress to environmental toxins.

Electrolytes

Electrolytes are chemicals that conduct electrical impulses when it's mixed with water. Electrolytes also regulate your muscle and nerve function and of course helps hydrate the body. It balances acidity in your blood and the pressure in your blood as well. It starts to rebuild any damaged tissue that your body may have experienced complex trauma through exercise. So, cells run on electrical impulses and they need plenty of electrolytes dissolved in water and in your diet.

Your cells that can carry on the electrical charge can communicate with one another. This means it's really important that they get the right amount of electrolytes in the water that you drink so that cells can do their job.

The different types of electrolytes that your body needs are Fluoride, Calcium, Magnesium and Potassium. Firstly, you can get these electrolytes through good quality foods and hydration, however, I'd always recommend to understand what levels of the electrolytes you currently have before you go down the route of adding supplements. Remember that supplements should be supplementary to your lifestyle, not something you depend on all of the time.

Hydration And Its Impact on Digestion

The quality of how well your foods are digested depends on the availability of adequate hydration. The journey of food from the mouth to the stomach, through the intestines, and eventually to absorption is deeply connected to how much water is actually present. Good, quality hydration makes sure that the smooth journey of nutrients helps digestion and the absorption processes that need to happen every single day.

In particular, the mucous lining of your gastrointestinal tract requires sufficient water to maintain its protective function. This barrier protects the gut from harmful substances, pathogens, and irritants. If you are not hydrated well and consistently every day, then this starts to compromise the protective barrier, potentially leading to gut inflammation, discomfort, and eventually digestive disorders. A well-hydrated gut serves as a resilient protector against digestive disturbances so that you can go about your day without any issues.

Not only that, hydration can influence your microbiome because good hydration supports the growth and activity of good bacteria therefore forming a really diverse and strong microbial community.

Dehydration on the other hand, flips the switch meaning it supports the growth of the bad bacteria which ends up disturbing the delicate balance of your gut also known as dysbiosis.

Cognitive and Emotional Balance

The Gut Brain connection is not just to do with digestion but extends widely out to how your brain cogs are turning and your emotional wellbeing and hydration plays a huge role in this.

Dehydration can affect cognitive performance, leading to difficulties in concentration, memory, and decision-making. This also affects productivity, focus and everyday activities. This also means, hydration plays a big role in our emotions too. It can create mood swings like feeling irritated, tension, anxiety all leading towards digestive discomfort.

Here are some practical strategies to consider with hydration and it require you being mindful and intentional in getting good quality hydration in:

1. **Listen to your body**: I used to say it to myself so many times that I must drink more water only to find myself saying it over and over again and never achieving the goal. The best way to really get into

the habit of drinking more water is looking at the colour of your urine first thing in the morning. Use this to set up the rest of your day of hydration no matter how quiet or busy it is. Signs like dark urine, a dry mouth and tiredness are good signs that more water is needed.

2. **Your Foods**: Eat foods that are rich in different types of fruits and vegetables in getting plenty of fiber in that work for you and many of them are high in water content like cucumbers, watermelon, oranges etc. It contributes to hydration and the health of your gut.

3. **Mark it**: Get a permanent marker and create small dashes down your bottle of water so that you can see how much you've drank and how much to go. Or just buy a bottle where the markers/prompts are already on there.

Realistically speaking, there is no magic hack of getting more water into your day other than being really intentional and mindful about it and actually wanting to do it. So, have a go at it and start putting reminders in your diary so that a good habit starts to form from here on. Deal?

Chapter 9
Gut Health And Movement

There is a hidden harmony between your gut health and how you move. The Gut as you know now is a complex system with trillions and trillions of microorganisms and is responsible for many functions. Not only does your microbiome influence and aid in digestion but also immune responses, brain health, metabolism and certain nutrients however the movement also plays a crucial role in shaping and balancing your microbiomes.

Research shows that regular movement has shown gut bacteria to be more diverse which creates this beautiful environment to support the good bacteria. The more diverse your microbiomes are, the more your body's ability to digest and absorb nutrients is better.

Let's view how you move your body like a dance. Every step you take in how you move your body creates a rhythm and this is a rhythm of movement that runs through your entire gastrointestinal system playing a huge role in maintaining healthy gut motility. It's the rhythmic movements that help your food move along the digestive tract. So, when you don't move much in a day and this is consistent throughout your year and you are quite sedentary, it can lead to sluggish digestive movements with a high chance of it leading to constipation and digestive discomfort.

Having regular movement activities in your day leads to better gut motility and bowel movements and it stimulates the muscles of the digestive tract which all in all makes the digestive system much more efficient overall.

Movement Vs Exercise

Just like your body changes with the seasons and your eating patterns change over time, so does your exercise rhythm as well over the years. In the last 10 years, I've done a fair amount of events and activities when it comes to exercise. I certainly have had my fair share of over-exercising, almost to a point where I was training seven days a week, sometimes twice in a day, all to sort of change my body shape and how I felt about my body at the time. Zooming out, it wasn't a very healthy way of moving my body and ultimately not the best way of helping my immune system along the way either. I did 5K to 10K runs to half marathon to a full one. The only thing that ever came out of that is my ego having a bring grin on her face and me realising how much I hate running. I've also moved on from running and picked up on cycling where I did charity bike rides doing hundreds of miles riding till I no longer could feel my legs. I enjoyed it more than running yet I didn't love it.

Then, I moved onto hiking, treks and mountain climbs. I've done some really strenuous climbs and treks, particularly when I've not really fully prepared my body inside out to handle that. So, my body didn't really have the capacity to even take that kind of exercise on and it just wasn't a healthy way of moving. However, I love it so I actually took the time to fully prepare my body inside out from food to clothing to hydration to sleep etc. I paid more attention to doing it properly. I do feel we are heavily pressured by society that we need to be doing exercise by being in a gym which isn't necessarily true.

I would encourage you to get your body moving first and see what it likes before hitting it hard with weights and exercise regimes. Just meet your body where it is sometimes. That's self-care and love at its best. Walking everyday from 10 minutes to an hour started to become my best friend from when I was recovering my gut infection back then and slowly increased it to more movement when I built up my immune system more and resiliency.

Healthy movement is about relieving stress and is the most caring thing that you can do for your body. Healthy movement is having no restrictions on how long you move for and just using your intuition to what your body actually needs that day or moment to moment. Healthy movement is taking a break from exercising, workouts and so on without the feeling of fear, anxiety, shame and guilt coming over you.

Healthy movement is all about being flexible with your workouts. Healthy movement is enjoying connecting with your body and how you feel every single day. Healthy movement is loving your body and what it does for you.

So, here are some practical strategies to consider with movement and helping you become more mindful and intentional in getting good bouts of movement in throughout your day:

1. **Schedule it in**: There's no such as not having the time so if it's not in the diary, it just won't happen. Set the intention to schedule whatever activity you want to do in your day. I usually like to use Sunday mornings to look at my week ahead and how my schedule looks with my business and my self-care.
2. **Get regular**: If you struggle to do any activity at all, then start with walking everyday for 5 mins and then generally build it up from there. This is how I started once I came out of clearing my bacterial infection. I had to take it easy and start building my

foundation from a different level. I then gradually build this up to 10,000 steps a day rather than time which is what works best for me. Start with 5 minutes a day and then gradually build yourself from there and get into a routine of what works best for you with your lifestyle and where most of your time goes.

3. **Hydration**: You know now how important this part is so no further explanation is needed here.

Chapter 10

Gut Health And Your Environment

You are the product of your own environment meaning your environment shapes you physically, emotionally and mentally.

So, my question to you is how clean is it? How clean is the quality of air you are breathing right now? What about the products you use on a daily basis? There's lots to consider…

Low exposures can just be as unstable and as unbalanced and just as dangerous as high exposure to your health, because you can be exposed to so many compounds in one go, which can dramatically change your health negatively. My biggest belief is prevention is always better than cure when it comes to how much toxic load is in your body. What I mean by this is can your body handle what it is exposed to?

Some common toxins that you probably have heard of or perhaps may have experienced the overload of it is:

- **Pollen**: Which can irritate your sinuses coming from the outside
- **Prescription Meds**: A bit of toxic cocktail mix which

causes all sorts problems to the immune system

- **Mould**: Produces allergens, irritants and sometimes toxic substances.
- Internal infections
- **Heavy metals**: Like arsenic, lead, mercury

So much of these toxins can cause Methylation problems. Methylation is all about how well you can operate physically and mentally.

As an example, Methylation is a bit like when you sit in your car, and you put the key into the ignition and you turn it and the car starts. You can turn on the radio, you can do the wind wipers, you can pull down your window, you can start steering the wheel and the car will move forward. Methylation is how your body gets the energy out to all the different types of systems in the body. So, you are exposed to certain things outside and inside, you can start to methylate quite poorly and then combining this challenge with an imbalanced gut bacteria, then you are in trouble with your health.

Now, you can't avoid toxin exposure because it's everywhere, however it's important to raise your awareness of your own surroundings.

Just take five minutes now and think about the area you live in and ask yourself what's close to your home? Are you near a main road or motorways? Are there fields nearby or massive telephone poles and buildings? Are you close to a lake, sea or river? Are there factories near or warehouses etc? It's worth just raising your awareness first.

Your emotional and mental state can also serve you and not serve you too. Your beliefs shape you whether it is negative or positive. Toxic relationships, being a people pleaser, being inflexible, a fixed rigid way of thinking, staying in your comfort zone for a long time end up being more intoxicating for you and your body than you can imagine. Your body is designed to adapt to changes as best as it can, yet if your emotional and mental state stays the same, then you develop a disconnect between your mind and your body and you then enter this crazy cycle of low energy thoughts, feelings and actions. You must become in alignment with yourself inside out.

As you now know that your gut is a protective fortress looking at harmful pathogens, pollutants and toxins that enter your body through ingestion, inhalation and absorption. Its role in doing this well is absolutely crucial.

Here are some practical strategies to consider when it comes to reducing toxin exposure:

1. **Nutrient-Rich Diet**: Eat whole foods rich in antioxidants, vitamins, and minerals that support the body's detoxification processes. Include cruciferous vegetables, berries, and herbs like coriander and parsley. Garlic, cauliflower and onions are really good at drawing out toxins and clearing them.

2. **Fiber Intake**: As I've mentioned in earlier when I spoke about Gut Health and its relationship with food, I would encourage you to start getting more fiber into your diet to support regular bowel movements, which aid in toxin elimination. Berries, whole grains, legumes, and vegetables are excellent sources of dietary fiber.

3. **Minimize Toxin Exposure**: Reduce exposure to environmental toxins by choosing organic foods, using natural cleaning products, and minimizing the use of plastics.

I love using Black & Blum and love using companies like Method and Neat for my natural cleaning products. Full transparency, I have no affiliation with these companies, I just think they are awesome.

I want to share an example of toxin exposure of a client me and team worked with back in 2021. Shantilal's life was just very stressful due to his ongoing health problems. He had been diagnosed with diabetes in 2011 and he was put on Metformin 500 mg twice a day as his blood sugars were constantly staying high and he used to get severe acid reflux because of the excessive food intake. His blood sugars kept on increasing at that time too so his Doctor increased his dosage of Metformin to 1000 mg twice a day. He had regular blood tests done annually but still didn't see a change in his blood sugars going down from the medications he was on.

He ended up in hospital on several occasions due to vomiting, as his small intestine was narrowed. He had to have a necessary stent operation on his small intestine so that it didn't collapse. It was actually one of Shantilal's daughters that arranged a meeting with me and my team back in Feb 2021. She has seen me and heard me on a podcast talking about Gut Health and thought to just reach and ask questions.

Whilst Shantilal was suffering with high blood sugars, he also had high blood pressure too which he was on medication for as well. He was carrying a lot of weight around the middle of his stomach, experienced bloating and was just low in energy.

Before he started working with me, he did have reservations and pushed back a few times which is completely normal to feel as all the help he had up until this point was with the National Health Service (NHS). He actually wasn't keen at the very beginning but it was his daughters that encouraged him to try The Gut Intuition approach. He just wasn't ready to fill in the forms in detail however he did in the end with the help of his wife and daughters. Having the right support around you goes a long way.

Now before Shantilal came to work with me, he was retired (still is), was living a sedentary life at home with his wife and had a loving supportive family around him (still does). His diet mainly consisted of home cooked Indian foods and he was vegetarian and still is so his diet was mainly carbohydrates and sweet foods and very little amount of proteins. He also had a habit of eating quite late as well.

My team and I spent a good amount of time getting to know Shantilal first and his lifestyle and this is an important part of the process which is listening with two ears and asking quality questions when speaking. It makes making changes for the long term a lot easier when you know their lifestyle.

In the first month of working me and my team, we looked at making some small changes to his diet and getting some blood tests done. Shantilal got this done via his GP and the results showed to no surprise that his blood sugars were high and he had low B Vitamins too.

As a collective decision, we decided that it would be best for Shantilal to have an Organic Acids Test (OATS) done with his B vitamins being low and knowing how many years he had spent working near an airport.

An OATS test is basically a urine test and is very useful to assess nutritional deficiencies that can affect someone's metabolic pathways. It's a great test to get a "big picture" of someone's health.

We got him a blood sugar monitor with strips as we knew he was diabetic. He pricked his finger up to 3 times per day to see how his diet impacted his blood sugar levels. It's a useful tool to determine someone's optimal diet. Nowadays, there are much easier and time savings methods to measure your blood sugars than the traditional finger prick test. This is also just another example of how personalised nutrition matters.

Test results always take some time to get analysed by the labs, put into a detailed lab report and then sent back to me and my team. However, the work actually started from our very first Zoom meeting and below are the followings steps that Shantilal started to implement slowly but surely into his lifestyle before his test results arrived:

1. **Eating Hygiene**: We got him to just monitor his meal timings for 7 days and we noticed he was used to having late dinners (after 8pm) out of habit, which had an impact on his blood sugars and digestion. So, with just a few small steps, we got him to just cut back an evening by an hour so he could eat his dinner by 7pm instead. We also got him to eat less heavier meals going from 4-5 times to 3-4 times a day instead.

2. **More protein**: By monitoring his food diary for 7 days, we noticed quite quickly that he wasn't eating enough protein, which is essential for cellular repair and energy, particularly for elderly people. Being a vegetarian, we got him to include more beans, quinoa, lentils and eggs to his diet gradually so that he could use it and stick to it more.

3. **Less caffeine and not on an empty stomach**: He was drinking a lot of black tea so we got him to drink less after food and not before.

4. **Less sweets**: He was eating a lot of biscuits between meals so we suggested a couple of swaps that had friendlier ingredients that weren't going to irritate the gut as well as much less sugar in it too such as Nairn's biscuits.

The above changes approximately took a good month to implement and stick to because let's face it, making changes is hard anyway so the best approach for Shantilal here was smaller changes and consistently and showing the reasons why that change needed to take place as well. After 3 to 4 weeks in, his test results were ready and this is exactly what it showed:

1. **Mitochondrial Dysfunction**: Shantilal had high lactic acid, which indicates poor conversion of carbohydrates into energy. Lactic acid builds up in the bloodstream when there is low oxygen delivered to muscle tissue (low oxygen was also another thing we picked up from his blood test). If lactic acid builds up in the body more quickly than it can be removed, acidity levels in bodily fluids spike which can contribute to high blood pressure and digestive problems. Also, if you have fluctuating blood sugar levels or long-standing diabetes, you are more prone to elevated lactic acid levels because of the difficulty delivering oxygen to active muscle tissue.

2. **Toxic exposure**: The test results also showed quite high exposure to toxins found in plastic, gasoline, pollution, preservatives and pesticides in foods, etc. This is highly likely due to spending many years in his previous job working near airports.

3. **Poor Methylation**: Firstly, let me explain what methylation actually is. Methylation is like a tiny chemical tag that your body uses to control many important processes. It's a bit like a light switch for your genes. When something in your body needs to be turned on or off, your body might add or remove these little tags through a process called methylation. This helps your body follow the right instructions and do the right things at the right time. Just like how you use switches to control the lights in a room, your body uses methylation to control how your cells work.

Methylation can influence how the body responds to insulin, the hormone that controls blood sugar levels. Poor methylation might affect insulin sensitivity, potentially contributing to insulin resistance. So, with Shantilal's high blood sugars, it's not surprising that methylation for him was quite poor.

4. **Candida overgrowth**: Candida is a yeast that is part of the intestinal flora and is usually harmless.

However, when you consume too many refined sugars, when you are also chronically stressed or sleep-deprived, or when you take a lot of medications, Candida can rapidly increase and it can cause symptoms such as sweet cravings, fungal issues, fatigue, anxiety, poor sleep, etc. Shantilal also had this issue at the time.

So, what happened next after we went through the test results? These were the steps me and the team advised him to take and start slowly implementing to start making even more solid changes to his lifestyle:

1. **Diet**: No more eating crisps after breakfast, to eat yogurt and cheese no more than once a week as this is a candida recommendation due to his overgrowth. Getting more protein in as he is vegetarian through pumpkin seeds, nuts, lentils, chickpeas, etc. At this stage, we did not go for any antimicrobial as it might have been too aggressive.

2. **Lifestyle**: We got him to really think about toxin exposure and it's a challenging one because toxins are literally everywhere which you can't avoid. However, we recommended filtering water and eating more organic produce to start the journey of reducing exposure to environmental toxins.

3. **Supplements**: Interestingly, we introduced two key
    supplements to help him and support the changes
    he was making. Firstly, we introduced Digestive
    Bitters because they promote healthy digestive
    processes and give support for a healthy digestive
    system, promoting digestive enzymes to encourage
    best absorption of nutrients from the foods he was
    consuming. This was three times a day and was in
    liquid form 10 minutes before every meal.

Secondly, we introduced Coenzyme Q10 (CoQ10) with
all the vitamins and minerals that he needed at that time
and he started with 1 capsule with a meal a day. CoQ10
is an antioxidant that your body produces naturally.
Your cells use CoQ10 for growth and maintenance[6]. If
you remember earlier, one of the first things that
showed up in Shantilal's lab report was Mitochondrial
dysfunction and mitochondria are the batteries in every
single cell of your body. A study by Dludla et al back in
April 2020 showed that CoQ10 may help reduce low-
density lipoprotein (LDL) cholesterol and total
cholesterol levels in individuals with diabetes, lowering
their risk of heart disease[6]. More research is needed
however some studies are showing some promising
results.

So, what was Shantilal's outcome after all these changes? Check them out below:

1. Within the first 2 weeks, he already had more energy which is something he flagged up before he started working with me and my team that he felt he was really low on. This continued to improve all the way through.

2. Healthier blood sugars: At week 1, his blood sugars were at approximately 9.8/10 and by the end of the 12 weeks, they were at approximately 5.5/5.8.

3. He had better digestion overall and this showed up as regular bowel movements.

4. He lost weight around the middle and as you can imagine was very happy about that. It's because he reduced as much stress and inflammation as possible with the new tools and resources he had gained over 3 months.

5. The most important part of all his journey was spending time with his family and having plenty of holidays away.

6. When he started working with us, he was on a medication called Alogliptin twice a day and this

was to control his blood pressure. His doctor stopped the medication because his blood pressure had gone down and he longer needed to take it anymore.

Fast forward to today, in his own words this what Shantilal had to say about his health journey:

"Since joining The Gut intuition back in 2021, I was given comprehensive plans for my diet with more protein based options and meals at regular times. I have controlled my blood sugars and the gut issues by following the plans introduced by The Gut Intuition team. I am more energetic and I stick to my regular diet and exercise plans to stay healthy and control my sugars. I still have to take Losartan to control kidney function but the diet plans introduced by Shim have helped me maintain my health. For that I have no regrets and would give 5 Stars ratings. In the end I am happy to have been introduced to Shim by my daughters".

What a beautiful and successful journey Shantilal had gone through and I hope by reading his story, it inspires you to know that there is always another way to get to the root of the issues.

Chapter 11

What Is Your Body Really Telling You?

H.E.A.L

In today's modern society, the word 'healing' has been thrown around a lot without ever truly understanding the meaning of it.

Through my life experiences, here's what I believe the word, 'Heal' stands for me:

Help: The journey of deep healing isn't meant to just be you by yourself being a martyr. It's about being brave and courageous and asking for help, the right type of help you need to reset, reboot and upgrade.

Energy: Energy is everything! Gaining a very clear understanding on what energy frequency you have been in can create positive and negative results, experiences and symptoms.

Action: Awareness is a fantastic place to start however that's where most people stay in what I like to call 'research/snooze mode'. Without taking any type of action, you will just stay in the same place but your body won't. I would recommend starting with Acceptance, Awareness and then Action.

Love: As fluffy as it sounds, for me love conquers all. You have to master how to unconditionally give love towards yourself and how to receive love towards yourself first. This is the one area that I had avoided a lot in my life simply to protect myself from getting hurt. Ever found yourself saying, 'well if you ever want to get a job well and fast, then you just got to do it yourself'?

Don't! It'll cost you a lot and I am not just talking about money.

Every human being on this earth has something they need to heal from situations that were perhaps out of their control and caused on some level trauma, disruption and damage.

Essentially, when it comes to healing, it doesn't mean that the damage never existed, it means that the damage no longer controls your life. So, it's the attachment you give to that damage. It's the identity you give, it's the energy that you infuse it in every day. Unhealthy attachments are formed such as you can't get over an ex, you can't get over someone that has done you wrong, abandonment, injustice, dismissal, or dismissive behavior. The more you feed it, the more it grows.

Remember, you don't get a physical problem because it's a physical problem, it goes way deeper than that. I visited a good friend of mine in May 2021 and she did a Kinesiology session with me. Kinesiology is holistic therapy which uses muscle response testing. She picked up some pain within my lungs and picked up on a lot of loss, heartbreak and grief; just layers and layers of things I hadn't fully addressed and it was physically and emotionally painful. It's amazing all the information that can be picked up on from one trigger/area of your body.

You don't need to hand over control of your health to anyone, not me, not a specialist or your doctor. It's your decision because it's your body. You have a gut intuition for a reason and that is your biggest protector in your healing journey.

Body Awareness

Awareness is the first step to understand what your body might be trying to tell you and start releasing unwanted stress from your body. Without it, you end up just feeding the same stress cycle over and over again. Scanning your body is a powerful technique to add everyday because it's an excellent way to release tension in areas you didn't realise you were experiencing. Sometimes, you can get so caught up with your stress that you may even forget the physical symptoms that your body is communicating with such as headaches, migraines, back, shoulder and neck issues to stomach discomforts. This is all connected to your emotional state as much as your physical state.

Some of the key benefits to being more body aware are:

- Allows your breathing to slow down & under control
- Calms your nervous system
- Helps release tension
- Increases your awareness of your own body quickly

How To Become More Body Aware

1. In a comfortable position either sitting or lying down, close your eyes and allow your breathing to come to a natural state
2. Starting at the top of your head, simply 'scan' down slowly your entire body
3. Move onto your neck, shoulders, arms, hands, chest, back, hips, stomach, legs, feet etc.

4. Start to take note if any of the areas you start to feel any sensations, feelings, discomfort
5. Take about up to 30 seconds on each area
6. If you find a particular area tight, has a lot of tension then simply focus on that area for longer and breathe a little more deeper; with each deep breath really releasing that tension.
7. Keep a pen and paper handy to make a note of any observations on any feelings, thoughts have come up
8. Remember, you are simply using this exercise to just be more present and get a good understanding of how your body is feeling

You can try this exercise every day and carry it out between 3 to 5 minutes. Give it a go!

Chapter 12
Why Does Disconnect Happen?

Healing ultimately is about working on the connection within yourself and to understand how you disconnect and where you disconnect and what you need to do to come back home to yourself again.

How people connect and disconnect is an area I am incredibly passionate about and it's why I do what I do when it comes to looking at your health inside out. I am like a female Colombo, a health detective who just won't quit or give up until getting to the root of the problem in a satisfactory way.

Here's my thoughts on why disconnect happens.

Firstly, let's split the word into two so it's dis-connect.

D - Desire

When you are not clear on what you desire in different areas of your life, results can become beige, lame and uninteresting.

I - Impact

Not making the impact you desired because the desire wasn't there in the first place therefore you may question if you matter in this world and whether you are making a difference.

S - Solutions

You did actually get the solution you wanted because the desire and impact just wasn't there.

When desire, impact and solutions are nonexistent, you end up trying to get to A to B without any clarity, desire, passion and guts. You become a hit and hoping champion and forever have your fingers and toes crossed that it will work out. Everything becomes surface level. This was in fact me many years ago, wanting to change my body shape without really understanding what the drive/desire was for changing my body shape; other than the fact that I just wanted to fit in more with the gym industry and follow the herd of what everyone was doing at the time.

You then fall into this pitfall of finding comfort through sugar, alcohol, sex, jumping from one relationship to another, exercising and feeding the unfulfillment then getting to grips of what you truly desire.

From my experience, the relationship between self-love, self-confidence, self-worth, and gut health is connected. The more I put my own needs first and gave myself the attention and care that I needed and rightly so wanted, the more the relationship with myself just improved daily. They were often little changes but consistently over time and that was the magic for me. The more self-care practices you have in place, the more positive impact it has on your gut health and overall well-being.

There is growing evidence that the more you practise self-love, the less stress and tension you experience which takes the pressure off of your gut, nervous system and overall your entire body. Self-love, self-worth, self-confidence comes down to choices, habits, boundaries, practises and beliefs in all areas of your life.

3 Ways To Reconnect Back To Yourself

Here are my top three ways that I have personally used often to reconnect back home to myself and feel free to start using one or two to begin with and then you will start to form your own ways for yourself that work for you.

1. **Spending Time In Nature**: It's become one of my favourite ways of spending time with myself, going

from daily walks in my local park to climbing mountains like Snowden, Scafell Pike, Ben Nevis at the weekends a few times to one day long distance hiking trails. This helps whether you live in the city and short on time to want to change your environment at the weekend and go and explore. Either way, all it requires is some planning and scheduling into your diary and away you go.

2. **Journaling**: I'll be really honest with you that when it comes to really addressing things that were frustrating me or just pissing me off, I would have had those thoughts just ruminating in my mind going round and round and simply giving me a headache. I had a lot of resistance to sitting down with a pen and paper and writing down my thoughts. I felt it was a waste of time and I had this belief that you don't solve anything by doing that. So many times over the past few years, the opportunity to journal came up for me but I never took it seriously. It wasn't until earlier last year that I really went for it and had the most deep insights and revelations to my questions that I had. I felt I bonded with myself a lot more and felt that I had created a lot more head space and emotional space within myself to be more creative because I dumped my worries onto a piece of paper. So, if you are

anything like me and there is resistance towards just writing it out, speak it out to yourself instead and just give it a go and respect the process.

3. **Reach Out To Someone You Trust**: Having a few good individuals who have got your back without judgment and just love you anyway is really key to reconnection. I am very grateful for the six months of counselling sessions I had with a counsellor to dig deep into some of my triggers that I felt were just controlling my life and how I viewed myself. It was very uncomfortable however it was a necessary part of my growth as the person I am today. I am also grateful to my business partners that I have to have those one to one times and just talk things through about business but also about personal stuff that sometimes affected how I ran my businesses and how well I looked after myself. I am forever grateful for those individuals who gave me their time and I was just able to talk things through and felt like I had a breakthrough every time.

Chapter 13

The Link Between Depression
And Gut Health

Depression is a widespread mental health condition affecting millions of people worldwide. It has become consistently evident that suffering with depression is a result of just your mind. It's actually also bringing in your environmental influences, lifestyle choices, how you fuel your body with food and drinks and what you are actually doing with your life meaning living with purpose and intent.

Around 1 in 4 adults in the UK will experience a mental health condition and 1 in 6 adults will experience anxiety and depression in any given week10.

Your brain and your gut are intimately linked meaning if your gut is in trouble and not well, it sends signals to the brain and vice versa therefore the stress causes more distress and anxiety overall because that's the signal/message that is going up and down your body.

Changes in your gut microbiome can have a huge impact on your mental health. As you now know from reading the chapters much earlier in this book, you know the role inflammation plays out in your body, particularly chronic inflammation. Imbalances in the gut microbiome can lead to chronic inflammation, which is increasingly recognized as a contributing factor in depression. An overactive immune response triggered by an unhealthy gut can affect both brain function and mood regulation.

You also now understand the role Serotonin and Dopamine play too so having an imbalance in microbiomes disturb these neurotransmitters and leading to more depressive symptoms.

Stress is a known trigger for depression, and the gut microbiome can influence your response to stress. A healthy gut microbiome helps regulate the body's stress response, reducing the risk of developing depression.

The most effective and easiest way to start improving your mood is with the foods you are eating. I want to give you some really easy suggestions on your food intake so that you can start to bring more diversity into your gut with different types of nutrient packed foods that will start to help bring back some balance into what you are consuming and how you are feeling.

1. Avoid processed and packaged foods because they have a lot of additives so are hard to pronounce and will disrupt your gut microbiome because they are in foods to prolong shelf life without much nutrients in them.

2. Get a range of fruits and vegetables: A range of different types of foods that are rich in nutrients, prebiotics and probiotics is really important to achieve balance with your food, mood and energy levels so I have put some examples below that are necessary for you to start including your diet slowly but surely.

Examples Of Plant Based Foods:

Watercress, spinach, beetroot, turnips, red, green and romaine lettuces, swiss chard, artichokes, leeks, beans, asparagus, fresh herbs like coriander, parsley, basil, rosemary, chicory greens, kale/collards, pumpkins, cauliflower, broccoli, brussel sprouts, red cabbage, butternut squash, papaya, onions, garlic, lemon, strawberries, blackberries, cherries, raspberries, blueberries, watermelon, pears.

Examples Of Meat Based Foods:

Oysters, liver/organ meats like spleen, kidneys, heart, poultry (giblets), clams, mussels, octopus, crab, goat, tuna, pollock, lobster, rainbow trout, salmon, snapping, herring.

The key thing to remember is having a balanced amount of seafood, lean poultry, a colourful range of vegetables and some fruits that are lower in natural sugars and consuming less red meat.

If you are a vegetarian or a vegan then definitely double down on more of the plant based foods with good quality supplementation to ensure you have plenty of vitamins and minerals available for in your body for necessary processes, enzymes etc to work to their fullest potential as well as a happy gut. It goes without saying that whether you are vegetarian, vegan or not, is to always ensure you are seeking expert advice on supplementation so that you are taking the right amount that is necessary for your body.

The link between depression and gut health is actually an exciting one that I feel is evolving over time. Gut-brain connection is becoming more and more evident and I am so pleased it's moving more towards a holistic approach as another way to prevent depression and other mental health problems.

Chapter 14

Work Life Balance Is BS!

The more you try to juggle this 50-50 balance between your job, career, business, health, life and relationships, the more the struggle of it can show up in your body too.

This is where Michelle was when she came to see me and the team back in 2022. She had major issues with bloatedness and just feeling tired. She just wasn't sleeping well and eating well either, waking up most nights at 3am.

The joy of eating foods she loved just wasn't there anymore and it knocked her confidence in wearing her favourite clothes too because it just didn't feel comfortable around her belly area anymore. She was suffering from bloatedness so much that she described it as that she looked pregnant for a slender woman.

Michelle is a busy business owner, International Best Selling Co Author, Professional Speaker and runs her own dental practice. She is very health conscious and she was already taking some good quality supplements too. She did work with a functional medicine practitioner in the past so she already had a good mindset around functional medicine and overall on her own health and wellbeing and that there is a link between gut health and oral health. Michelle also does Yoga and meditation and eats really well and also has a personal trainer.

Now you might be wondering that Michelle actually is really healthy and ticks all the boxes when it comes to her health so she shouldn't really be having any issues right? Not quite!

She tried to exercise more to reduce the bloating and tiredness but it didn't help at all and she started to feel like that she had to now live with this problem which really drained her and almost feeling defeated because she felt like she was doing all 'healthy' things like eating well, taking her daily supplements, got herself a Personal Trainer, doing daily Yoga and meditation but something still wasn't quite right.

Back in 1992 -2000, Michelle was actually diagnosed with Irritable Bowel Syndrome (IBS) but she managed to reverse the situation with proper hydration and fibre amongst other things. Fast forward to 2022, it was the bloating that was the main issue which sometimes lasted for hours on end even without consuming any foods.

The functional test we got Michelle to do was a 3 day Comprehensive stool test. This is a great way to assess someone's gut health. It can provide valuable insights into the root cause of gastrointestinal symptoms, as they can evaluate infections, allergies, digestive problems, inflammation, and more. Given that bloating was her main concern, me and the team suspected an imbalance of gut bacteria but we needed to see which bacteria were overgrown so we could create a custom plan to eradicate the overgrowth. It's important to never assume things because there can be lots of things, however this is the beautiful work of functional tests in getting to the root cause of gut issues.

Now while Michelle's lab tests were being analysed, we got her to tighten up her eating hygiene as she used to have late dinners (after 8pm) because of her workload with her dental practice. Eating late also meant she was going without having properly digested her meals. This increases the likelihood of having undigested foods in the small intestine, which make the perfect dinner for bugs in the large intestine. She carried on taking her supplements which were benfotiamine, zinc, selenium, vitamin E, reishi mushroom, liposomal Vitamin D3, N-Acetyl-cysteine.

Michelle's test results came back and this is what it showed us what was really going on at the time:

Maldigestion: Her body had a poor breakdown of protein and fats so she wasn't absorbing proteins and fats very well.

Dysbiosis: She had overgrowth of commensal bacteria which is bacteria that should be in the gut. So, the bugs are not necessarily bad however they are overgrowing, which disrupted the natural balance of her gut microbiome.

Methane Dysbiosis Score: Methane is a by product of bacterial fermentation. Now her test also showed an increase in Bacteroides, Odoribacter, Prevotella, Methanobrevibacter smithii, all of which are associated with methane production. Methanogens love to feed off hydrogen produced by other bacteria (they convert it into methane). The overgrown bacteria in your gut feed off of undigested food in your small intestine, specifically carbohydrates. This feeding process ferments the carbohydrates and produces hydrogen gas as a byproduct. Symptoms may include abdominal pain, loose stools diarrhoea, constipation, food allergies, headaches, and brain fog and the big one which is bloating and distention. In other words, methanogens slow gut motility and causes a lot of gas, bloating and constipation

So, what happened next?

We decided together to focus more on improving gut motility and eradicating the overgrowth of methanogens. She was already doing quite well anyway so here's the framework we got Michelle to follow to start bring her body back to a balanced state that works for her and not against her:

Diet: Eating healthy was something Michelle was already anyway however we focused on supporting digestion and gut motility first. We got her to use more natural antimicrobial herbs and roots in her cooking such as garlic, cinnamon, oregano, thyme etc.

Eating hygiene: Eating late even if it was a healthy meal was a factor we needed to address quickly. So, we advised Michelle to eat her dinner before 8pm to support full digestion or light dinners if it was after 8pm.

Improve gut motility: We also got her to limit her meal windows to every 5 hours so in other words, no snacking but just healthy meals.

Regular bowel movements: Methane Dysbiosis can cause constipation so having regular bowel movements can be a struggle most days. We introduced linseed/flaxseed tea for her to take one cup a day in the morning to see how her body responded and how her bowel movements changed.

Supplements:

Biofilm buster: Often, bacteria hide behind a biofilm and build resistance to antimicrobials, so it was important to start by destroying the biofilm before attacking the microbes with herbal antimicrobials. We got Michelle to take 1 capsule 2x a day.

Herbal antimicrobials: We also got Michelle to supplement with a herbal blend with neem, allicin in garlic and oregano to address the overgrowth of methanogens. She took 1 capsule a day.

Digestion: We also got her a blend of Hydrochloric Acid (HCL) pepsin, pancreatic enzymes and ox bile to support digestion. HCL is gastric juice which plays an important role in creating the right PH level for Pepsin activity. She took 1 capsule 3x a day with her meals.

So, what were Michelle's results from making all the changes?

Within just a few weeks, she didn't just reduce her bloating, she got rid of her bloating by 100%. This was a great sign that her body was craving for these holistic remedies and that they responded really well. Not only did she get rid of her bloating, she also felt an increase in her energy levels coming back, she had regular bowel movements so her gut motility improved, she felt more clear headed which is really crucial in decision making and with running her own business and a team to look after. The number result I absolutely loved when working with Michelle was her confidence came back in wearing her favourite clothes and her ab muscles peeking through again. Most people end up spending loads of money on just buying a new wardrobe because the clothes don't fit anymore however, Michelle knew that something was off in her body and she was determined to get to the bottom of it.

Now me and my team are a bunch of health detectives obsessed with getting to the root of digestive issues. Looking back at Michelle's lifestyle and healthy actions she took on a daily basis, she also drank Kangen water. This is basically hydrogen water and the idea is that the water is alkaline water to bring the body out of an acidic state and more into an alkaline state. It's my belief that the daily consumption of Kangen water was a big contributor to her digestive issues. This is a great reminder following health trends isn't always a good idea. Just because it's classed as 'healthy', doesn't mean it's going to be good for you and your body. My advice to you is to figure out your own 'balance' of your own body first and not get shiny object syndrome on the latest health trends and hacks that are out there.

Fast forward to today, what has Michelle kept up with after a year? This is what she had to say in her own words

"Today I can eat what I love, wear what I love and not look like I am pregnant and feel more confident in myself and the clothes and feel comfortable after meals. I am more aware and knowledgeable on how to manage it and eat earlier to avoid late night meals and reduce my intake to smaller meals and balance my diet - more fiber and less sugar. I am a conscious eater now and will continue in this manner to avoid gut issues. I am pleased with the outcome for my long term gut health stability - Thank you for your professional care and advice".

Chapter 15

Not One But Two

I'll never forget the day my mum came down the stairs and into the living room showing me the itchiness across her chest. It was a lovely summer's day around July 2019. She had developed some very mild itchy skin on her legs a few years back which seemed to have calmed down with a steroid cream. However, the steroid cream stopped working and the itchiness now spread across her upper body and she was getting a little worried.

My mum, Jasu, was my first ever client for The Gut Intuition. I was so grateful that a close family member of mine asked me to help them. You see, from experience people that are family or close friends never seek advice from you even when they know you can help them, just a weird thing that I've never really understood. However, helping my mum with her health was an absolute honour and a pleasure to work with. There were many times after my dad passed away that I wished I could have done more to help, maybe he could have lived a little bit longer but I realised and had accepted that it was what it was.

My mum had gone through a lot since the passing of my dad because a year after, she also lost her sister in law to whom she was very close with from where my mum was born and raised in Uganda to settling in the UK in the 70s'. So, when she started working with me and my team in August 2019, I was very aware of her emotional and mental state at the time but I loved her attitude of wanting to change her health and actually taking a different approach and to support me in my business too.

Not only did she have itchy skin all over but she was quite bloated most of the time. She felt like she was putting on weight, and felt uncomfortable in her own skin. When it came to her diet, it mainly consisted of homemade Indian food with vegetable curries and lentils with chapatis. Now, what was also really concerning her was that her gums were swelling up every time she ate anything a little spicy. For her, spice is life and she's had it all her life however, something wasn't adding up.

The first thing we did as a team was really look at her diet and get her to monitor what she was eating for all meals and snacks and take her blood sugar measurements and monitor this too; after all diet and blood sugars go hand in hand. Mindfulness eating was key for her to properly chew her food more, eat with no distractions around so that she could solely focus on her food.

Jasu actually needed help in all areas of her health foundations. Over the course of 3 months, we got her to eat more fiber and more protein so introducing eggs into her diet, we worked on stabilizing her blood sugar even more, better sleep hygiene because she was going to bed in the evenings quite late as well so switching off an hour before bedtime starting to make a huge difference in her energy levels. She had to wean herself off tea and balance her hydration out more with water to help her with focus, energy and all round good health. She also came on walks with me too every day to get her body moving; staying at home all of the time just kept reminding her of my dad so it was good to get out and about. I loved those walks together because we really helped each other at a deep, sad time in our lives and just got into remembering happier times about my dad, we spoke about the past a lot and reflected, we planned our holidays and of course we spoke about poop a lot too. It's hard not to when your daughter is a gut health expert, haha! It was tough for her to make all these changes because she had lived her life a particular way and the last big change her body went through was coming to England in the 1970s'.

We got Jasu to do a 3 day comprehensive stool analysis test. What we found out was she had not one but two parasites living in her gastrointestinal tract and they were Blastocystis spp and Endolimax nana. Such fancy names for parasites that can cause a lot of damage to you.

The presence of any parasite within the intestine generally confirms that the individual had come into contact with the organism through fecal-oral contamination. The damage parasites can often do to the person is blockages, pressure, immune inflammation, hypersensitivities and reactions, generally adding toxicity to cells and playing a role in the morbidity of these diseases. Acute parasitic infections can result in symptoms like diarrhea with mucus and sometimes without, blood, nausea, fever or stomach pain. If it's left untreated, parasites can cause damage to the intestinal lining and cause illness and fatigue.

Chronic parasitic infections can also be associated with increased intestinal permeability, irritable bowel syndrome (IBS), irregular bowel movements, malabsorption, gastritis or indigestion, skin disorders, joint pain, allergic reactions, and decreased immune function.

In all honesty, any type of gut related issue shouldn't be taken lightly.

I remember Mum's face on the call when we went through her results. She thought we were talking in a different language; I guess Gut health can be sometimes. She also had an overgrowth of Candida too which can grow when excess cortisol release is going on. Now, this wasn't a short term quick fix, a one size fits all approach, to a shit diet plan downloaded off from Google or a calories in to calorie case. The beautiful thing was, we didn't start her journey with her twiddling her thumbs waiting for her test results to come out, we got her stronger with the foundations of her health first so that she had the best chance of clearing these parasites out of her body. She had started working with us mid Sept in 2019 and by late October, her itchy skin had gone, the uncomfortable bloating and burping after meals had gone, disrupted sleep had gone too and energy crashes were a thing of the past and she hadn't fully finished working with us yet. The other brilliant results she got also was her hair was stronger, she was able to eat foods that once gave her a lot of challenges, and she lost half a stone too.

The whole process from start to finish was a combination of:

- Mindset
- Education of whole foods
- Listening to her body, her emotions and thought patterns
- Functional testing
- Herbal remedies
- Movement
- Blood sugar management
- Sleep hygiene
- Reducing stress
- Support and Accountability

and more.

Our approach for Jasu was in four phases which were:

Phase 1: Optimising digestion and detoxification
Phase 2: Parasite cleanse
Phase 3: Fungal clearance
Phase 4: Gut repair

We introduced the following supplements:

- **Enzymedica Digestion**: Helps to optimise digestive capability and function. It's quite potent digestive enzyme and has been formulated to assist in digestion of proteins, fats, carbohydrates and fiber. She was taking 1-2 capsules with each meal.

- **Triphala**: Cleanses and supports the entire GI tract, improving digestion and elimination helping in having healthy bowel movements. 1-3 capsules before bed

- **Swedish Bitters**: To stimulate digestion, settle the stomach before eating and neutralise. It can help Fight sugar cravings, relieves gas, bloating, flatulence, cramps and nausea. Increase digestive enzymes, bile & hydrochloric production. Jasu diluted a small amount of Swedish bitters in water and drank this solution 15 minutes before every meal.

- **CoQ10**: CoQ10 Has powerful antioxidant properties in the human body. Its activity supports the body's healthy response to everyday oxidative stress. It also plays a critical role in mitochondrial function of the cells, so absolutely crucial for energy production.

- **Support LV**: To support the Liver and Gallbladder and is designed to support bile flow for the normal processing and elimination of toxins through the specific combination of nutrients and herbs. Between 1 - 3 caps waking up

- **GI Microb X**: Is a blend of botanical extracts with a long history of use for supporting a healthy gastrointestinal microbial balance. 1 -2 caps waking up and before bed.

With all our clients, it was important to know what medications their doctor had put them on so that monitoring was always going on at all angles through the journey as well as working with other medical professionals too.

It's safe to say, Jasu did extremely well on her journey of clearing and repairing her gut. I remember we were on the plane to Gran Canaria in Dec 2019 and she turned around and just explained to me how comfortable she felt on the flight for the first time ever because she always struggled with stomach flare ups. Just hearing this made me so happy and I rest assured her that it was her that showed up for herself through grief, was open and coachable and gave it a good go no matter what and that actually has been why all my clients that I've had the pleasure of working with have had true success with their health. I do remember my mum turning around and saying to me during the pandemic that had she not asked me for help, her health would have been very different during Covid and she would have had a big fight for her health on her hands because of her immune system being down due to the parasites and Candida overgrowth.

For me, helping my mum in all areas of health was a true honour and a time spent with her that I'll never forget.

In her own words today, this is what she had to say about the experience with me and my team:

"I would say your wealth is your health. The Gut Intuition team was very helpful, polite and helped me in every way possible. Within 3 months, I was out of my problems which my GP couldn't help me with. The medicine that my GP provided was just for the time being, but The Gut Intuition got to the root of it. I'm so happy now with my health and have kept up with my timings around eating my meals, drinking water, sleeping, walking and doing a bit more yoga and stretching. God bless you".

Conclusion

Is The Clock Ticking?

Perhaps from reading this book, it may have triggered you, made you angry, you may have disagreed with some things, perhaps it has restored hope and faith that you can be healthy in your own way. Whatever it is, you got this far because it's given you direction and information that you never knew before.

I hope you have gained the awareness that your mind, body and soul are inseparable; that you have full permission to stop splitting yourself into different sections as you are not separate, you are actually whole. I hope this book has given you inspiration, insights and knowledge to start making better decisions and changes when it comes to your health. It all starts with you. Healing is a choice, not an easy one because it takes work to turn it around. However, the better choices you make for yourself, it can only ever go up from here.

The one thing that has been apparent in all the beautiful people I've had the pleasure to work with over the years is always work on your foundations of your health at all times and making it a non-negotiable. Why? Because you my friend are important, you matter and you deserve the best health on this planet that's clear, personalised and brings out the best of you.

I would encourage you from here on to stay connected and check out the resources and references page and you will find a lot more information I've gathered for you to check out in your own time.

Remember, being healthy isn't something you go out and get, health is something that you already have IF you don't disturb it.

Because before you know it, life will come in when you least expect it and change it…

Just like that…

About the Author

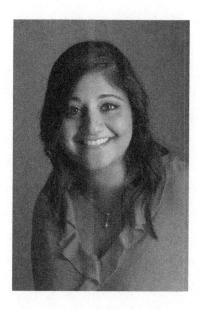

International speaker, number one best-selling co-author and gut stress expert, Shim Ravalia is the Founder of The Gut Intuition and Co-Founder of Queens In Business. With over 15 years of experience in Sports Therapy, Nutrition and Health, Shim helps highly driven entrepreneurs go from rundown and stressed to razor sharp focus so that they can continue creating their legacies without burning out. She has helped thousands of people get to the root cause of their health challenges inside and out using her unique approaches to reducing stress. Since running her very first business from 2012 -2018, Shim hit burnout many times to a point her health took a toll by the end of 2018. Since then, her focus and beliefs have been that health always comes first. Through the success of The Gut Intuition, Shim is on a purpose led mission to break the BS that is often taught about our wellbeing and giving individuals the right information and transformative tools to live well inside out.

Shim has been featured in the likes of NBC, ABC, Fox, CBS, Business Woman Today, Thrive Global, Authority Magazine, Ticker TV News, MSP News Global as well as best-selling book series The Art Of Connection and Queens In Business. Shim has also been featured on more than 50 different podcast shows including The Self Made Series with Bianca & Bryan Miller Cole, iNetpreneur, and Brilliance Business. In recognition of her outstanding contributions, she has also won the 2023 Greater London Business Awards in the Best Health & Wellbeing Facility category.

References and Resources

1. How much is the health food industry in the UK worth today:

https://oaknorth.co.uk/blog/the-success-behind-the-healthy-snack-market-science-and-data/#:~:text=Well%2C%20between%202016%20and%202021,trillion%20US%20dollars%20by%202026.

2. How much fructose sugar the small intestine can handle in healthy subjects:

Rao SS, Attaluri A, Anderson L, Stumbo P. Ability of the normal human small intestine to absorb fructose: evaluation by breath testing. Clin Gastroenterol Hepatol. 2007 Aug;5(8):959-63. doi: 10.1016/j.cgh.2007.04.008. Epub 2007 Jul 10. PMID: 17625977; PMCID: PMC1994910.

3. The Dopamine Reward system:

https://www.snexplores.org/article/explainer-what-dopamine

https://neuroscientificallychallenged.com/glossary/
mesolimbic-pathway

4. Sleep: Blue and Green Light

https://onlinelibrary.wiley.com/doi/full/10.1002/jbi
o.201900102

5. Hydration:

https://www.bulletproof.com/diet/healthy-
eating/how-to-hydrate-properly-cells/

6. CoQ10 lowering diabetes and risk of heart disease:

Dluda PV, et al. The impact of coenzyme Q10 on metabolic and cardiovascular disease profiles in diabetic patients: A systematic review and meta-analysis of randomized controlled trials. Endocrinology, Diabetes and Metabolism. 2020; doi:10.1002/edm2.118.

7. Gut Health & Immunity:

https://www.sleepfoundation.org/physical-
health/how-sleep-affects-immunity

8. People suffering with IBS in the UK:

https://transform.england.nhs.uk/key-tools-and-info/digital-playbooks/gastroenterology-digital-playbook/remote-monitoring-of-patients-with-small-intestinal-bacterial-overgrowth-IBS-and-food-intolerances/#:~:text=An%20estimated%2013%20million%20people,impact%20on%20quality%20of%20life.

9. The Emotion code resource:

https://richardmoat.com/

10. Depression Statistics:

https://championhealth.co.uk/insights/depression-statistics/#:~:text=Around%2017%25%20of%20adults%20in,presents%20significant%20challenges%20for%20organisations.

Printed in Great Britain
by Amazon

37076531R00086